EQUITY CHOICES AND LONG-TERM CARE POLICIES IN EUROPE

Equity Choices and Long-Term Care Policies in Europe

Allocating resources and burdens in Austria, Italy, the Netherlands and the United Kingdom

AUGUST ÖSTERLE
Department of Social Policy
Vienna University of Economics and Business Administration

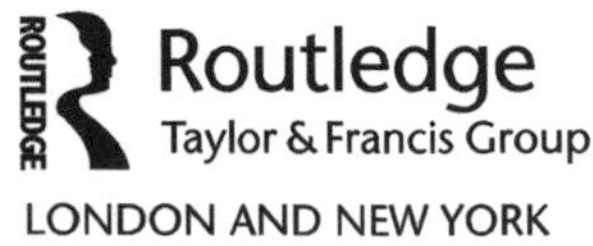

LONDON AND NEW YORK

First published 2001 by Ashgate Publishing

Reissued 2018 by Routledge
2 Park Square, Milton Park, Abingdon, Oxon OX14 4RN
711 Third Avenue, New York, NY 10017, USA

Routledge is an imprint of the Taylor & Francis Group, an informa business

A Library of Congress record exists under LC control number: 2001093277

ISBN 13: 978-1-138-63397-1 (hbk)
ISBN 13: 978-0-415-79146-5 (pbk)
ISBN 13: 978-1-315-21227-2 (ebk)

Contents

List of Tables

List of Figures

Acknowledgements

Many people have contributed to this book. I am most grateful for their time, their help and their advice. The idea for the study on equity in long-term care was originally born when I was a research fellow at the School of Social Sciences, University of Bath in 1995. Staying there was financially supported by the EU Human Capital and Mobility Programme and the Austrian Science Fund. It did however take some time to really work on the idea. Participation in the 1998/99 programme of the European Forum at the European University Institute in Florence on 'Recasting the European Welfare State: Options, Constraints, Actors' supported by the European Commission (DG V) has given me room to write major parts of this book and to discuss the issues in a unique interdisciplinary and international environment. Thanks are due to Maurizio Ferrera and Martin Rhodes, directors of the 1998/99 programme, and the distinguished group of academics I met there who created an intellectually stimulating environment. Staying there was financially supported under the Jean Monnet Fellowship Programme. Brief study visits to the countries covered in this book and a one-month stay at the London School of Economics and Political Science in September 1999 (funded by the EU Training and Mobility of Researchers Programme) have further contributed to the comparative study as have many people supporting me with comments or providing me with specific information such as Marja Pijl, Clare Ungerson and Christiano Gori. In its final stages, work on the book was undertaken at the Department of Social Policy at the Vienna University of Economics and Business Administration. Comments by Christoph Badelt, Head of the Department, Karin Heitzmann, Elizabeth Scharpf and Elisabeth Hammer have been most helpful to omit mistakes and to further improve the book. Many thanks to my colleagues at the Department. You make work a challenging experience but at the same time real pleasure. Thanks are also due to Katherine Hodkinson, my editor at Ashgate Publishing. The accuracy of facts and analysis remain entirely my responsibility.

August Österle

1 Introduction

It is only recently that long-term care became a major social policy issue in all welfare states. The debate on how to redesign long-term care policies is shaped by an increasing demand for care, changes in formal as well as informal support systems, changing values and attitudes towards informal care-giving and the division between private and public responsibility, as well as incentives and challenges from the social, political and economic environment.

Parallel to the novelty on the top-agenda of social policy, long-term care is one of the less researched areas in social policy. Long-term care has often been equated with care in nursing homes, reflecting the fact that public expenditure primarily was directed at this type of care setting. In recent times, parallel to the emphasis on care in the community, long-term care is more often equated with social services for the elderly. Although important, both aspects only represent parts of the wider long-term care issue. Apart from the provision of in-kind services, some countries nowadays regard payments for care as the key to their long-term care systems. In most countries there is a slow growing awareness of the gendered issue of informal care-giving, regarding long-term care policies not just as an approach to support those in need of care but also those who informally provide an often enormously burdensome amount of care. Overall, considerably less emphasis in research has been put on the long-term care system as a whole, which is even more true for cross-country comparative research.

Only in the 1990s was there an increase in comparative research on long-term care. The OECD produced a series of publications on the topic (e.g. OECD 1998; 1996; 1994) and the EU addressed the issue in the European Observatory on Ageing and other research activities (e.g. Pacolet, Bouten, Lanoye, Versieck 2000; Bettio, Prechal 1998; Walker, Guillemard, Alber 1993). A number of comparative studies looked at long-term care systems (Martin 2001; Brodsky, Habib, Mizrahi 2000; Eisen, Mager 2000; Rostgaard, Fridberg 1998; Weekers, Pijl 1998; Tester 1996; Giarchi 1996; Hugman 1994; Jamieson, Illsley 1990). Other studies focused more specifically on payment for care programmes in long-term care (Weekers, Pijl 1998; Evers, Pijl, Ungerson 1994; Glendinning, McLaughlin 1993), on home and family care (Hutten, Kerkstra 1996; Baldock, Ely 1996;

Leseman, Martin 1993; Jani Le-Bris 1993; Jamieson 1991), on gender issues in care (Ungerson 2000; Knijn, Kremer 1997; Ungerson 1995), on employment and care relationships (Naegele, Reichert 1999; Naegele, Reichert 1998; Phillips 1995) or a variety of specific economic questions (e.g. contributions in Eisen, Sloan 1996). Many of these studies include detailed descriptions of the respective elements in national long-term care systems, offering a valuable basis for any further research. The necessity of a multi-disciplinary and multi-dimensional approach in comparative work is widely accepted, but in the realisation only at the beginning. Efforts in cross-country comparative research have been hindered by considerable policy variations amongst and within countries, problems and constraints in data availability and comparability, as well as the lack of conceptual and analytical frameworks considering the specific characteristics of long-term care. The latter issue of missing analytical tools is one of the themes addressed in this book.

In this study the issue of long-term care is brought together with equity, which is at the core of welfare state and social policy definitions. Equity has been a central theme of the welfare state from the outset. And equity is an attractive label in social policy making. On the other hand, equity is still described as an 'elusive' issue. Approaches in analysing equity and even the definitions of equity vary considerably across and even within disciplines.

Searching for equity studies in long-term care is an almost fruitless task, although there are exceptions such as Evandrou, Falkingham, Le Grand, Winter (1992), Bebbington, Davies (1983) or most recently Davies, Fernández, Nomer (2000) and Davies, Fernández, Saunders (1999). However, most of the few existing studies address very specific interpretations of equity, other studies are locally restricted, or include only one type of service provision within the complex arena of long-term care. Although the concept of equity or equality is introduced in a number of studies, it is rarely based on an explicit specification of what is meant by equity or an equitable allocation. If there is such a specification, the choice of a specific interpretation often seems to be based on a mixture of what is supposed to be a widely accepted interpretation and what is going to be testable, given the data available.

Taking the broader perspective at equity studies in social policy one can identify three main streams of equity research: those studies analysing social policy issues in the light of theories of social justice, empirical studies investigating social justice perceptions and judgements, and those studies testing specific interpretations of equity (see part 3). The first line of normative research is very much theoretical with very little links to empirical studies. The second approach is focusing on justice beliefs and judgements with regard to allocation and distribution of resources and burdens on different levels of society. The third line of research has created a substantial amount of knowledge regarding the outcome of allocational procedures and the distribution of various resources with respect to specific interpretations of equity. What is widely ignored in research, is the way equity is translated into practice, the wide range of interpretations of equity that are used in practice. '... there have been virtually no attempts to study the whole range of questions of this kind, and to develop a conceptual and theoretical framework to describe and explain how institutions allocate goods and burdens.' (Elster 1992: 2)

With the focus on concrete situations, the 'empirical rules of equity' in long-term care and the way resources and burdens are allocated, a number of questions arise that will be addressed in this study: What does equity in long-term care mean? What are the relevant dimensions in equity interpretations? What does equity look like in actual long-term care policies? How does the state intervene in the allocation of long-term care services? How are payments for care distributed? How does the state allocate the burdens of financing long-term care? What are appropriate approaches to address these questions in a comparative perspective? How do different equity interpretations fit with basic equity objectives of the welfare state? What are the consequences of different approaches on care receivers? What are the impacts of different equity rules for informal care givers?

Regarding the research topic of 'Equity and Long-Term Care', two major gaps in research have to be identified: First, there is a lack of conceptual and analytical frameworks for a comparative study of long-term care issues. Second, there is a lack of equity research focusing on the variety of equity approaches to be found in practice. This study attempts to reduce these gaps in social policy research and to contribute to a better understanding of long-term care and equity issues in a comparative perspective.

Research questions and methods

By bringing together the social policy issues of long-term care and equity, the objective of this study is to comparatively analyse long-term care policies in Europe with regard to equity choices and to contrast the respective choices in selected countries with basic equity objectives in the welfare state.

The *theoretical objective* of this study is to contribute to the understanding of the rules and interpretations of equity to be found in long-term care policies by developing and conceptualising an analytic framework for the comparative study of equity choices in long-term care policies. 'Choices' here terminologically point to the wide array of possibilities and potential decisions that can made in the policy process to pursue the objective of equity. The focus here is not on the process but on the outcome of the process and herewith the design of long-term care policies with regard to equity. At the same time, choices that have been made are an important input for the actual provision, consumption and finance of long-term care. As suggested by the term 'long-term care policies' rather than 'long-term care', the focus is on the role of the welfare state in designing the long-term care system.

This concept requires a theoretical and conceptual consideration of long-term care as well as equity. As for long-term care, a clear definition of the concept and the content of long-term care is required to clarify the potential role and the objectives of the welfare state in long-term care. In order to systematically examine equity considerations in long-term care policies, the institutional and policy mix in long-term care has to be unpacked.

The equity focus of this study is on equity as a social policy objective, on how public policies interfere in long-term care systems by providing, financing, and regulating long-term care in terms of equity. It is not the objective of this study to analyse the normative question of how equity should be defined in long-term care or to analyse one specific interpretation of equity in long-term care, but to develop a framework covering the range of interpretations of equity.

Traditionally, categorisations according to welfare state principles such as universality vs. selectivity or social rights vs. social insurance vs. social assistance are used in this context. This is, for example, a convincing approach in searching for welfare state clusters or welfare state families, showing similar features across social policy areas. It does not, however, provide us with a clear picture of whether or not and to what extent equity objectives are promoted in single policy areas. Therefore, this study develops a different approach allowing a more thorough analysis of equity issues. The study will follow three basic characteristics according to which equity choices or interpretations of equity may differ: what is to be shared (that is the kind of goods to be shared, be it resources, benefits, burdens, costs, etc.), among whom (that is the subjects of the allocation procedure), and how (that is the principles according to which goods are allocated).

As mentioned before, equity research in social policy has been very much concentrated either on the analysis of social policy issues in the light of theories of social justice or the evaluation of outcomes with regard to very specific interpretations of equity. Both these approaches widely ignore the broad range of equity interpretations to be found in the design of welfare states. And this, in fact, is the focus of the study. It attempts to develop an analytical framework and to use that framework to investigate how public policies intervene in the allocation of resources and burdens in long-term care. Furthermore, the analytical framework offered here represents a helpful tool not just for the empirical study undertaken within this project but for future research on equity issues in long-term care as well as in other areas of social policy.

The *empirical objective* of this study is to contrast equity choices in different European countries with basic equity objectives in the welfare state. It will be studied whether or not and to what extent actual allocation policies are promoting these equity objectives. The countries selected are Austria, Italy, the Netherlands and the United Kingdom. These countries are generally regarded as representatives of very different welfare state models with regard to objectives, design and outcome. At the same time they share a cultural and socio-economic context and major social and economic challenges to the welfare state.

Explicitly or implicitly, welfare state definitions and social policy definitions include notions such as equity, justice or equality, they are even at the core of these definitions. Equity is widely accepted as an objective in social policy and is an attractive label in social policy making. However, apart from a basic agreement on equity as an objective of the welfare state, we are far from reaching an agreement on what constitutes equity. Precise specifications of equity are rare. There is no common clear-cut definition of equity as a welfare state objective. The study, therefore, will use a set of equity objectives underlying the concept of modern welfare states.

Whether or not and to what extent these objectives are promoted in the countries selected will then be tested by investigating how public policies intervene in the regulation, provision and finance of long-term care. Here, the analysis follows the framework developed in the theoretical and conceptual part of the study. The empirical analysis of the actual choices made in the design of long-term care policies is divided according to the provision and the finance of long-term care. Considerable attention will be paid to the role of informal care givers and how they are addressed by long-term care policies as in-kind financiers of long-term care.

It will be shown that equity choices that are found in the design of long-term care policies in different countries are characterised by a complex mix of objects, subjects and principles of allocation. This complexity tends to be hidden by basic principles of welfare design, used, for example, in various attempts to categorise welfare states. In the final chapter, the potential and the comparative advantage of equity choices as a conceptual tool for studying welfare policies will be discussed.

Before proceeding, three methodological remarks seem necessary to place this study in research on welfare state and social policy issues.

The study is characterised by an interdisciplinary approach. Social policy, and given the institutional and policy mix, even more so health and long-term care issues, are prime examples for topics that are situated at the cross-roads of various policy areas. Long-term care policies are closely interrelated with health policy, demography, family policy, labour market policy, broader issues in social policy, economic policy, etc. And health and social policy are situated at the crossroads of the various streams in the social sciences. In the design and its basic idea, socio-economics can be seen as the background of this study. However, by choosing equity and equity choices as the object of the analysis it is focused on an issue whose coverage is rather limited in economics. This becomes obvious by looking at any textbook in economics or sub-field of economics, although there are prominent exceptions as theories of justice developed by the economic science or distributional issues in public finance.

It is regarded as an adequate approach to explicitly place this study at the crossroads of the social sciences. This has, as in all forms of research, both potential and problems. It does not restrict itself to a single methodological approach, but is characterised by incorporating elements from different disciplinary approaches. This cross-sectional pluralism is an appropriate approach to study pluralism in social policy in general, and in long-term care in particular.

Any interdisciplinary approach implies the question of what terminology to use. Equity and related issues are a prominent example that terminology differs quite considerably between disciplinary approaches, and – in that case – even within disciplines (see chapter 3.1). Using the term 'equity' in accordance with, for example, economics might well be in contrast to using that term in the context of political science, sociology, law or any other social science. This is true for many of the terms that have to be used in this study. It is hoped that with the study proceeding clarifications regarding terminology will help to overcome potential misunderstandings.

Finally, with regard to the comparative empirical study, there is the question of data and data quality for cross-country analysis. This will be discussed in more detail in chapter 4.1. As will be shown, due to constraints in data availability and comparability, the approach of the empirical study has to be qualitative as well as quantitative (based on secondary data) and to a considerable extent of exploratory nature.

Summing up, the study has theoretical and conceptual as well as empirical objectives. The theoretical aim of the research is to contribute to a better understanding of equity choices in long-term care and to conceptualise relevant dimensions of allocating resources and burdens in a framework for systematic comparative analysis. Based on this analytical framework, the empirical aim of the study is to map and to systematically compare long-term care policies in Europe with respect to equity choices. The results will then be contrasted with welfare state objectives and discussed in a broader welfare state context.

The structure of the book

Apart from this introduction the book is divided into five main parts, each of which is introduced by an overview giving an outline of the objectives and the methods of the respective parts.

Part 2, 'Long-Term Care and the Welfare State', represents an analysis and conceptualisation of long-term care and long-term care policies in the context of the welfare state. This part is introduced by an overview of the various aspects that recently made long-term care a major social policy issue. (*chapter 2.1*) These developments include an increase of long-term care needs (due to the so-called ageing of society), changes in formal as well as informal support systems and incentives from the social, cultural, economic and political environment, such as changes in values and attitudes towards informal care-giving, the division of responsibilities between the private and the public sphere, the implications of social security and labour market regulation on the provision of informal care or the debate on financing the welfare state. *Chapter 2.2* will then be looking at the concept of long-term care, developing a working definition for the analysis to be undertaken in this book. Because the usage of this concept enormously varies in research as well as in social policy practice, some restrictions in the empirical analysis will have to be made, as will be shown in more detail in *part 4*.

Part 2 continues with an investigation of long-term care and the long-term care system. In *chapter 2.3* the long-term care system will be analysed by looking at the production and the consumption of long-term care as well as the mix of actors and policies involved. It is aimed at the development of a 'map' which then can be used to evaluate different policy approaches in long-term care in a cross-country perspective. Finally, *chapter 2.4* will be investigating efficiency, good merit and distributional issues as potential arguments for welfare state intervention in long-term care.

In *part 3*, 'Equity and Long-Term Care: A Framework for Analysis', the concept of equity will be introduced, and dimensions and interpretations of equity will be systematically specified and discussed with regard to their relevance for long-term care. The analysis follows the distinction between the provision of long-term care focusing on care receivers, and the finance of long-term care focusing not only on monetary contributions, but particularly on informal care givers in their role as in kind contributors. After the introduction, some terminological and methodological preliminaries will be made in *chapter 3.1*. As will be shown, there is an enormous range of very different approaches to the concept of equity across and even within research disciplines.

Chapter 3.2 presents different approaches to the study of justice and equity. Apart from the basic ideas, it briefly surveys the respective literature on long-term care related issues, showing a lack of attempts dealing with equity concerns as they are translated into social policy design. The basic structure of this study will be introduced in *chapter 3.3* by discussing the main features of equity choices and placing the study in equity research. The object of allocation (what is to be shared?), the subject of allocation (among whom?) and the principles of allocation (how?) are identified as key characteristics of equity choices and further developed as an analytical tool in *chapters 3.4* and *3.5*.

The conceptualisation of equity in the provision of long-term care is undertaken in *chapter 3.4*. The allocation of burdens, that is the finance of long-term care, will be analysed in *chapter 3.5*. Here, particular emphasis will be put on the role of informal care givers, which all too often is completely neglected in the analysis of the finance of welfare state measures. Recognising this form of in-kind contribution will also highlight the gendered issue of informal care-giving.

In *parts 4 and 5* the analytic framework developed in part 3 will be used for a comparative empirical analysis of equity in long-term care policies in four European countries: Austria, Italy, the Netherlands and the United Kingdom. Whereas most equity studies in social policy attempt either to search for *the* interpretation of equity, or to analyse one specific interpretation of equity, the objective of this part is to search for and to analyse the range of equity interpretations in long-term care systems and to contrast these choices with basic equity objectives in welfare states. The focus is on the allocation of resources (provision) and burdens (finance) through public policies.

Part 4, 'Investigating Long-Term Care Policies in Europe', is introduced by a discussion of comparative analysis in long-term care in *chapter 4.1* addressing approaches of cross-country analysis, discussing possibilities and constraints arising from variations in definitions and concepts as well as the availability and comparability of existing data. Following this discussion and the objectives of the study, Austria, Italy, the Netherlands and the United Kingdom are selected for the empirical study. In *chapter 4.2* equity as a welfare state objective will be introduced. Starting from various attempts to categorise welfare states and to define equity objectives, a set of equity objectives is identified against which choices to be found in the four countries will be studied. *Chapter 4.3* gives an overview to long-term care policies in Europe, as well as more detailed information on long-term care in Austria, Italy, the Netherlands and in the United Kingdom.

The actual comparative examination of equity choices is undertaken in *part 5*. The comparative investigation of equity choices in the provision of long-term care *(chapter 5.1)* and in the finance of long-term care *(chapter 5.2)* follows the three main features identified in *part 3*, that is the resources and burdens to be shared, the focal units among whom these resources and burdens are allocated, and the principles of allocation. It attempts to capture convergencies as well as differences in the four countries with regard to these features. In the concluding *chapter 5.3* the spheres of provision and finance are brought together and equity choices are contrasted and discussed with regard to basic equity objectives in the welfare state. In the concluding *part 6* of the study, results and prospects will be summarised and discussed in a broader welfare state context.

[illegible] Investigating Long-Term [illegible] Policies in Europe', is introduced by a discussion of comparative analysis in long-term care in [illegible] and addressing approaches of cross-country analysis, discussing possibilities and constraints [illegible] variations in definitions and concepts [illegible] the [illegible] and comparability of existing data. Following [illegible] Sweden, Italy, the [illegible] for the empirical study [illegible] welfare [illegible] will be introduced. Starting from [illegible] identified [illegible] which [illegible] four countries [illegible] (Chapter 4) [illegible] long-term care policies [illegible]

[illegible]

2 Long-Term Care and the Welfare State

Long-term care is a most heterogeneous social policy field. Long-term care is provided consistently over an extended period of time and contains medical as well as social services; the bulk of long-term care is delivered within informal, in particular family networks; the extent and structure of formal private and public support varies considerably between countries; the division of responsibilities between the various actors in the formal and the informal sphere often leaves considerable room for discretionary interpretation. On the social policy agenda as well as in social policy research, long-term care is often equated with parts of the whole long-term care issue or restricted to specific subgroups of the population. Altogether, a systematic analysis of the different concepts of addressing and organising long-term care and a thorough understanding of the characteristics of this policy field is indispensable for any further analysis of equity issues in long-term care. The focus of this part of the study is on the general construction of long-term care systems. Reference to specific countries is made for the purpose of illustration. Long-term care systems in Austria, Italy, the Netherlands and the United Kingdom will then be looked at in more detail in parts 4 and 5 of the study.

The objective of this part of the study is to unpack and to analyse the concept of long-term care and the institutional and policy mix that might be found in long-term care systems. The section is introduced by a chapter on the growing importance of long-term care (chapter 2.1). This will underline the dimension of the long-term care issue and the kind of developments, challenges and constraints societies are facing in the design of long-term care systems. Then the diversity of approaches to define long-term care and the target group of long-term care policies will be analysed in chapter 2.2 to establish a working definition for this study. 'Welfare pluralism' in long-term care will be analysed in chapter 2.3. Starting from a model of the production and consumption of long-term care, this chapter looks at institutions and policies that constitute a long-term care system. For conceptual reasons a division will be made between the sphere of providing and the sphere of financing long-term care. With regard to the overall objective of the study, this part of the study finally addresses the question as to why the welfare state might intervene in long-term care. Efficiency, good merit, distributional as well as public choice issues and the valuation of these issues are key determinants for the extent and the design of welfare state intervention (chapter 2.4). The main conclusions of part 2 are presented in chapter 2.5.

2.1 The growing importance of long-term care issues

The 1980s and the 1990s have been characterised by considerable changes in the design of the welfare state (see e.g. Esping-Andersen 1996; Pierson 1994). For the 1990s this is also true for long-term care. However, whereas other welfare state reforms were very much caused by financial pressures and aimed at cost-containment and increasing efficiency, the driving forces of changes in the long-term care systems seem to be more diverse. Except for the Nordic countries, the Netherlands and to some extent the UK, long-term care was primarily a social assistance issue. Only in the 1980s and increasingly in the 1990s, the development of home and community care, the quality and appropriateness of care, the cost and funding of care and the support of informal care are reported as major policy concerns in all OECD countries (Kalisch, Aman, Buchele 1998). Although responsibilities are still put heavily on family and other informal networks, long-term care is increasingly regarded as a social risk where an effective, equitable and efficient balance between private and public obligations is sought.

Behind the various policy concerns there are at least four sets of arguments that brought long-term care to the top-agenda of social policy. The reasons are the following:

- demographic changes regarding the number of people (potentially) in need of care,
- changes in the traditional support systems and the role of informal care-giving,
- social, political, and economic factors influencing the structure of production and consumption, and
- the overall economic situation and the question of macro-efficiency.

The development of long-term care needs

Long-term care needs arise from physical and/or mental limitations. Potentially, everyone might be effected by such limitations at some point in his or her life, elderly as well as non-elderly people. However, as elderly people are most likely to need long-term care and because of the so-called 'ageing' of society (see e.g. Kobayashi 1997), a considerable increase in long-term care needs is expected in this age group. Before presenting some key figures an important remark has to be made: It is highly misleading to regard 'ageing' just as an increase in dependency. As will be shown below, elderly people are at the same time an important resource in care-giving in the long-term care system.

Table 2.1 Demographic information

Country	Population aged 65 and over (% of total population)			Population aged 75 and over (% of total population)		
	1990	2010	2030	1990	2010	2030
Austria	15.1	18.3	25.7	7.1	8.3	11.6
Belgium	15.0	17.1	24.3	6.7	8.2	10.9
Denmark	15.4	16.4	22.6	6.7	6.6	10.4
Finland	13.3	16.2	24.1	5.6	7.3	12.1
France	13.8	16.3	23.3	6.5	8.1	11.4
Germany	14.9	20.2	28.1	7.2	8.4	12.4
Greece	14.2	19.0	24.6	6.4	9.3	11.8
Iceland	10.6	12.0	19.6	4.3	5.5	8.6
Ireland	11.4	11.9	16.4	4.6	5.1	7.4
Italy	14.8	20.6	27.9	6.5	9.9	13.4
Luxembourg	13.6	17.3	25.6	6.0	7.6	11.5
Netherlands	13.2	16.4	26.0	5.6	7.2	12.1
Norway	16.3	15.8	23.0	7.0	7.7	11.2
Portugal	13.0	15.0	20.9	5.2	6.7	8.6
Spain	13.2	17.6	24.9	5.4	8.6	11.2
Sweden	17.8	18.4	23.1	7.9	8.6	12.1
Switzerland	15.0	19.1	27.5	7.1	8.7	13.6
United Kingdom	15.7	17.0	23.0	6.8	7.9	10.6

Source: OECD (1996)

The majority among those people in need of long-term care are frail elderly people, with the 'old elderly' being most likely to need long-term care. And the number of people in this age-group has been rising considerably and will continue to increase. In 1996 11.7% of the EU population (57 million people) were 65 years of age and over, 3.8% (14.5 million) 80 years of age and over. The share of those 80 years of age and over ranges between 2.6%

in Ireland and 4.7% in Sweden (Eurostat 1997). In OECD Europe the share of the population aged 65 and over to total population will have more than doubled between 1960 (9.7%) and 2030 (23.2%). The share of those aged 75 and over to total population will increase from 6.0% in 1990 to 10.8% in 2030 (OECD 1996) (For further details see Table 2.1.).

What is common to all EU countries, and in fact all other industrialised countries, is a substantial growth in the number of elderly people, which tends to lead to a growth in the number of dependent older people in the coming decades. Whether or not and to what extent there will be a growth in dependency among elderly people not only depends on the age structure, but on the probability that elderly people will be affected by limiting health conditions. This is expressed by the *long-term care dependency ratio*, with dependency referring to physical and/or mental dependency and the consequences regarding needs for support. The dependency ratio is calculated by dividing the number of dependent people in a certain age-group by the total number of people in this age-group.

Because of enormous variations in the approaches to define long-term care dependency across and even within countries (see chapters 2.2 and 4.1), it is an almost impossible task to give a clear-cut picture of this dependency ratio. According to the European Community Household Panel the proportion of people hampered in at least some activities well increases the 10% share. This however does not necessarily require an extended support by others or even welfare state intervention. This can be illustrated by another figure: In Austria 4.0% of the population receive payments for care (BMSG 2000). This programme is based on a quantitative as well as qualitative definition of long-term care restricting public support to those with care needs of at least 50 hours per month (For further details see chapter 4.2).

There is no consensus among experts, whether or not and to what extent the dependency ratio will change as a consequence of higher life expectancy and progress in medicine. There are three different theories to be found – the expansion of morbidity thesis, the compression of morbidity thesis and the dynamic equilibrium thesis – all of which are supported by empirical work (Cambois, Robine 1996). According to the 'expansion of morbidity thesis' (Olshansky, Rudberg, Carnes, Cassel, Brody 1991) there will be an increase in chronic diseases as a consequence of longevity and the postponement of death. The 'compression of morbidity thesis' (Fries 1980) suggests that the period of long-term care needs will be compressed if the time when morbidity occurs can be postponed. Finally, Manton (1982) argues that higher life expectancy and a decline in mortality will increase chronic diseases. These, however, will be less severe than they tended to be ('dynamic equilibrium thesis'). Based on a review of the literature and recent trend studies, Cambois and Robine (1996) support the thesis of an increase in light and moderate disabilities, but not of severe disabilities.

As with regard to consequences, even if a decline in the prevalence of disabilities is assumed, there will be an increase in the absolute number of people in need of long-term care because of demographic trends. Varying prevalence ratios would cause considerable variations in the extent but not in the general direction of an increasing demand for long-term care.

For Austria, it is estimated that among those 60 years of age and older the number of people in need of long-term care will increase by 64% between 1990 and 2030, assuming constant dependency ratios. Under the assumption of an increase in dependency between 0% and 20% for different elderly age groups between 1990 and 2030, the number could almost double (+ 95%). In a better health scenario – here dependency ratios are reduced by between 10% and 35% for different age groups for the period 1990 until 2030 – the decrease in dependency probabilities would still mean an increase in the number of dependent elderly people by 31% (Badelt, Holzmann, Matul, Österle 1996). For Germany, for the period 1995 – 2030, it is estimated that the number of people in home care will increase by 26.7%, those in nursing homes by 43.9% (Schmähl, Rothgang 1996). An even sharper increase is forecasted by Schulz, Leidl, König (2001). Their study suggests that the number of people in need of care will increase by 52% between 1999 and 2020, and could more than double till 2050. Similar trends are reported for all industrialised countries (e.g. Mayhew 2000; Manton, Corder 1998; Grundy 1995; Manton, Corder, Stallard 1993; Laing 1993). In another recent study, projections for selected countries on the development of dependency rates are combined with institutional arrangements, with one projection assuming stable rates of dependency, and a second projection based on observations available in the respective countries (Jacobzone, Cambois, Chaplain, Robine 1999). Overall, both projections – although not homogeneous for different countries and different subsets in the population – show an increase in disability. For some countries (France, Sweden) a slight decrease is estimated for disabled elderly people living in the community for the period 2000 - 2020. As for the consequences, these studies point at two issues: Firstly, there is an important role for social and health policies in influencing epidemiological trends. Focusing on prevention and activation might considerably reduce disability rates. Secondly, care arrangements and the balance of different institutional settings plays a most important role for the quality as well as the economic impact for the future of long-term care.

Support systems in long-term care and the role of informal care

The lack of a predetermined finishing date and unpredictability of the intensity of care needs make long-term care a social risk with quite considerable effects on those in need of care as well as informal care givers. Though, against what might be expected, public support in long-term care has been rather limited compared to other areas in social policy – with the exception of the Nordic countries, the Netherlands and to less extent the UK.

The bulk of care-giving was and still is predominantly done unpaid in the informal sector. Even for the Netherlands – where a comparatively high level of social service support exists – it is estimated that the number of hours spent in the informal sector is eight times as high as in the formal home help sector (Kwekkeboom cit. in Rostgaard, Fridberg 1998). For the UK it is estimated that the value of informal care is at least five times as high as the value of formal care (Glendinning, Schunk, McLaughlin 1997). In an OECD Europe estimation informal long-term care represents at least three quarters of the value of care (OECD 1994). Although there are considerable variations in the figures, the general trend is common to all the calculations. This is even true for Nordic countries characterised by a high level of social service supply. In Denmark as well as in Sweden, in more than half of all caring relationships it is a person within informal networks that acts as the main care giver. The respective figures reported for these two countries are 56% and 67%, respectively (Hennessy 1997). In other countries the share of private informal care is considerably higher. In Austria, informal carers act as the main care giver in 80-85% of all care relationships, another 10% are cared for in institutions, in the remaining 5-10% a formal service supplier is seen as the main carer (Badelt, Holzmann-Jenkins, Matul, Österle 1997). According to the Austrian microcensus 1998 (with regard to care for elderly people for more than a week) 70% are cared for within informal networks, whereas care by social services accounts for 14%. For the remaining 16% there is either no care available or answers were missing (Badelt, Leichsenring 2000). For France it is reported that 90% of care outside institutions is undertaken by informal carers (Hennessy 1997). In Italy, 88% among those living at home are cared for by family members, another 9.8% by a combination of care-giving from the informal and the formal sector (Taccani 1999).

The majority of informal carers acting as main care givers are women caring for their parents, parents-in-law or their partner. Among women, those between 40 and 60 years of age tend to be most committed to care). About 80% of the main care givers are women, 20% are men most of whom are caring for their spouse when they are retired (see e.g. Schneekloth, Müller 2000; Badelt, Holzmann-Jenkins, Matul, Österle 1997). Other studies suggest that the number of men providing long-term care is higher (e.g. Clarke 1995; Sundström 1994; Fisher 1994). At the same time – and apart from the question of different response behaviour between men and women – these studies also support what was stated before: women are more likely to take the main responsibility in care-giving, women spend more hours on long-term care-giving, women are much more likely to be a care giver for people other than the spouse, and they offer care before retirement age and herewith face the question of whether and how to combine formal employment and informal care. These sharp gender differences in informal care-giving are to be found in all European countries (Bettio, Prechal 1998).

Carers under the age of 65 are facing the problem of balancing work in the regular labour-market and care-giving. A considerably higher proportion of male carers tends to be in formal employment alongside providing informal care than women. Whereas men are almost exclusively in full-time employment, a considerably higher proportion of female carers in formal employment are part-time employed. Joshi (1995) reports for the UK that more than half of those carers in formal employment are working part-time. In Austria, labour market participation of carers tends to be smaller, but among those participating in the labour-market only one third is working part-time (Badelt, Holzmann-Jenkins, Matul, Österle 1997). As shown by a number of studies, informal care-giving does not produce a significant reduction in formal employment as long as informal care is restricted in the number of hours (e.g. Ettner 1996; Wolf, Soldo 1994). Participation in the regular labour market is however reduced among those who provide long hours of care. According to Carmichael, Charles (1998) the threshold is 20 hours per week of informal care work. Despite the limited effect of informal care-giving on hours of formal employment, the studies show considerable opportunity costs (Carmichael, Charles 1998; Ettner 1996). Apart from a slightly reduced number of hours per week, combining formal work and care-giving results in lower earnings per hour, reduced opportunities regarding future career opportunities, as well as negative effects on social participation, family relationships and health.

The number of elderly people acting as main care givers for frail elderly or handicapped people is often ignored. Elderly people are far from being just the target group of receiving care, but a most important resource, including care-giving (George 1996; OECD 1988). This is supported by various studies. It is estimated that on average only five out of one hundred in the age group 60-69 are severely disabled, whereas the proportion increases to about 30% among those aged 80 years and older (Walker, Alber, Guillemard 1993). On the other hand, a rather high proportion of elderly people are care givers. According to Arber, Ginn (1991), 35% of total care is provided by people aged 65 and over, in the case of co-resident care almost half of total care. In Austria, 37% of the main care givers are 60 years of age and over. Consequently, elderly people are not just those in need of care, but those who offer an enormous amount of care for other people. Higher life-expectancy and postponing morbidity could even further increase the potential of this resource.

Regarding the future design of long-term care systems, the question about the availability of an informal 'care-taker pool' (Moroney cit. in Sundström 1994) has to be faced. The care-taker pool, that is the potential of informal long-term care-giving resources, is determined by a number of factors. First of all, there is the question of co-residence and solitary living. A number of studies have shown that informal care-giving is more extensive in the case of co-residence (e.g. Clarke 1995; Kemper 1992). Living in private households with close relatives, makes these relatives – in particular partners and daughters or daughters-in-law – to informal care givers. And the bulk of long-term care-giving is mostly done by only one person. Over the last decades, there was a considerable increase in solitary living and a decline in co-residence (Sundström 1994). In the 1990s, in many European countries one-person households represent more than a quarter of all households, in Denmark even 45%. In more than half of all single households the householder is 65 years of age and older in Southern Europe as well as the United Kingdom and Ireland, whereas the elderly age-group represents between 30% and 40% of the single households in the other countries (see Table 2.2).

Increased solitary living (and related expectations or attitudes) require different responses in long-term care. Solitary living does not necessarily affect the existence of informal long-term care-giving, but will tend to reduce the number of hours provided. Higher mobility in the population will make it even more difficult to provide long-term care. Requirements from the labour market organisation regarding flexibility might work in both directions, offering opportunities to adapt working time to caring responsibilities as well as reducing such opportunities by the necessity of flexible availability.

Marital status and the rate of childbirth are seen as another indicator of the informal care-taker pool. Higher rates of divorces, a smaller number of children per family and higher rates of childlessness as realised in most European countries (see Ditch, Barnes, Bradshaw, Kilkey 1998; Saraceno 1997; Hantrais 1994) may tend to reduce the number of close relatives acting as informal carers. However, there is less of an effect of these changes in family patterns on the present generation of people to be cared for, than on those who will be in need of care in the second or third decade of the 21st century and onwards (Clarke 1995).

Table 2.2 Solitary living in Europe

	One-person households (% of total households)	One-person households with householder aged 65+ (% of one-person households)
Austria	29.7	46.4
Belgium	28.1	43.9
Denmark	44.8	39.0
France	28.0	42.1
Germany	33.9	38.6
Greece	19.5	49.8
Ireland	21.7	51.2
Italy	22.2	55.2
Luxembourg	26.0	36.9
Netherlands	32.5	38.0
Portugal	13.5	62.2
Spain	12.8	58.5
United Kingdom	27.8	53.9

Source: Ditch, Barnes, Bradshaw, Kilkey (1998); ÖSTAT (1999)

A third argument determining the informal care-taker pool is the rate of employment participation. As most male informal carers, at least in their role as main care givers, are retired, this affects particularly women. However, the assumption that a higher rate of employment participation means a reduction in the amount of informal care-giving is not supported by empirical studies (e.g. Joshi 1995; Arber, Ginn 1995; Phillips 1994). There seems to be no significant impact on employment participation up to a limited amount of hours of informal care-giving per week. But, the higher the number of hours spent on informal care-giving, the more conflicting formal employment and informal care-giving there becomes. People who spend long hours of informal care-giving per week (from about 20 hours per week) tend to be just part-time employed or have to withdraw completely from formal employment. This trend is to be found for informal care givers providing co-resident care as well as informal care givers providing non-resident care (Arber, Ginn 1995). Apart from the care-giving task, decisions whether to withdraw from the formal labour market on that occasion seem to be determined by a number of additional factors, such as having been in very low paid periphery employment, their own health status, etc. (Sundström 1994).

Overall, an increasing rate of employment participation – as realised all over Europe (see Table 2.3) – does not necessarily mean a proportionate decrease in the number of care givers within the family. Care givers, mostly women, find or have to find arrangements – sometimes supported, sometimes enforced by public policy measures – to care for a close relative even if this person does not live in the same household as well as arrangements to combine formal employment and care. Those women who spend long hours of informal care-giving tend to work just part time or to withdraw from formal employment. In any case, informal care-giving tasks tend to be very burdensome. Most carers face a huge amount of total work hours per week, either because they have to combine formal employment and informal care-giving or they have to provide long hours of care. In addition, withdrawal from as well as reducing formal employment to part-time work, has considerable negative consequences regarding income, career opportunities and the position in the social security system (see e.g. Watson, Mears 1999; Holzmann, Österle 1996; Arber, Ginn 1995; Phillips 1995; Hooyan 1990). These effects tend to become even more problematic with the increase of entitlements derived from formal employment alongside trends in long-term care policies to reinforce care at home. Long-term care policies, therefore, will have to pay considerably more attention on the situation of informal care givers and on what terms formal employment and informal care-giving are combined (or have to be combined) (Watson, Mears 1999; Naegele, Reichert 1998; Doty, Jackson, Crown 1998; Phillips 1995; Hoskins 1993; Neal, Chapman, Ingersoll-Dayton, Emlen 1993).

Evidence suggests that long-term care systems are not faced with an immediate decline in the number of people offering informal care-giving, but a decrease in the amount of time spent on informal care-giving. For the future, given changes in family and household patterns and in the socio-economic environment, long-term care systems more recently promoting care at home will increasingly be faced with a further reduction of informal care offered in the community.

Table 2.3 Labour force participation and part-time employment

Country	Part-time employment [1] (% of total employment)		Female labour force participation (%) [2]	
	women	men	1988	1998
Austria	22.8	2.7	53.7	61.9
Belgium	32.2	4.9	51.2	57.8
Denmark	25.4	9.8	77.6	75.3
Finland	13.0	6.7	73.0	69.9
France	25.0	5.8	57.1	60.2
Germany	32.4	4.6	55.4	63.1
Greece	15.4	5.3	43.5	-
Iceland	38.6	9.8	68.0	81.2
Ireland	31.2	8.2	37.6	52.6
Italy	22.4	4.9	43.2	45.0
Luxembourg	29.6	2.6	47.2	-
Netherlands	54.8	12.4	50.6	62.7
Norway	35.9	7.9	72.8	76.3
Portugal	15.8	5.1	58.2	65.2
Spain	16.6	2.9	39.6	47.8
Sweden	22.0	5.6	80.1	72.6
Switzerland	45.8	7.2	58.0	70.3
United Kingdom	41.2	8.2	63.7	67.2

1) Part-time employment defined by a common definition of less than 30 usual-hours worked per week.

2) Female labour force of all ages divided by female population aged 15-64.

Source: OECD (2000)

This leaves the question: To what extent are formal private or public services able to compensate for this potential decline? (For a detailed description of the long-term care system see chapter 2.3.) Institutional care – at least as it has been designed in the past – tends to be a substitute for informal care-giving, but there are considerable changes under way. For efficiency reasons long-stay beds in hospitals were successfully reduced in many countries. This and other factors led to a considerable increase in the number of beds in nursing homes. These institutions in turn also had to reduce the number of beds or to concentrate institutional care on those with severe care needs. For those with more moderate care needs, care in the community or semi-residential care-settings (such as day centres or sheltered housing) are favoured (Hennessy 1997). Semi-residential care settings as well as domiciliary care are not just a substitute for informal care-giving, but to a considerable extent a complement. As will be shown in more detail in the empirical part of this study, this role as a complementary element in the system is becoming even more important with other recent reforms. Increasingly, the availability of informal care-giving is – explicitly or implicitly – taken into account in the assessment of care needs. Formal care-giving tends to be concentrated on those with more severe care-needs and limited or no informal support (see chapter 4.3).

Social, political and economic factors determining demand and supply

All these changes in the support system described above are determined and influenced by a number of different factors to be found in the social, the political and the economic environment: values and attitudes towards informal care-giving and family obligations, expectations, as well as incentives and disincentives from the design of welfare state policies.

First, whether or not and to what extent long-term care is offered within the family or within households is a question of values and attitudes towards the role and the responsibility of families and family members in a given environment (Millar, Warman 1996; Leat 1990; Finch 1989). As shown by Finch (1989) and Finch, Mason (1993) there are quite considerable differences in what people perceive as family obligation, what they actually do when they are faced with a situation that requires care-giving, and how the design of welfare state policies intervenes in the decisions to be made. Intra-family decisions regarding family care are the result of a complex interrelation of issues such as altruism, reciprocity, reputation, autonomy, traditional forms of labour division, the emotional relationship between family members as well as the influence or the perception of external issues discussed below.

Parallel to an increase in solitary living (not only in old age), independent living became an increasingly important issue. In long-term care the concept of independent living choices is mostly connected with handicapped people. But there also seems to exist a strong and increasing preference among elderly people not to co-reside with their children and, in the case of care-needs, not to be cared for by someone within the family. There is no systematic evaluation regarding the question, whether or not and to what extent this follows or precedes the development of formal provision of institutional care and social care in the community. But, there is a remarkable parallel development of public services in long-term care and the acceptance to receive such care (Sundström 1994). This suggests that in those countries where domiciliary care services have been developed only recently or will be developed more widely in the near future, will also realise an increase in the demand for such services.

In a number of countries long-term care for close relatives is legally defined as a family obligation (Millar, Warman 1996; Twigg, Grand 1998). Many countries have in practice withdrawn from this obligation long before they have abandoned the legal obligation or they practice this obligation in a way that reduces the financial responsibility to co-payments. On the other hand, there also seems to be a tendency to reinforce the actual obligation of families, be it by increasing co-payments or by including the availability of informal support in the assessment of needs (Millar, Warman 1996; Rostgaard, Fridberg 1998).

The connection between the expansion (or reduction) of the welfare state and the perception of what is seen as welfare is an important issue. An increase of public support in long-term care creates rising expectations in the role and the responsibility of the state in long-term care. But it is not just state intervention in the long-term care system that determines expectations in the community regarding long-term care. The ability and the willingness to provide informal care is determined by a number of issues in related policy fields, as for example the response of the traditional social security system to changing family patterns. Welfare state policies do not only affect the policy field they are aimed at, but they do create a number of incentives outside this sphere. Herewith, the success of the welfare state in one sphere might create challenges to the welfare state in another sphere, what then often is misunderstood as a failure of the welfare state (George 1996; Prisching 1996).

For example, with regard to social security, recent welfare state reforms attempt to reinforce the relation between social benefits and participation in the labour market (re)introducing entitlements derived from employment participation. Given the increase of divorces, the declining number of children per family and the increase in solitary living, this supports the reduction of intra-family arrangements regarding social security, and creates considerable economic incentives to participate in the labour market. Whereas the approach might be strongly favoured for reasons of economic performance as well as from a gender-equality perspective, it also creates new challenges for the welfare state.

As shown above, an increased participation in the labour market does not necessarily mean a reduction in the availability of informal care-giving.

But it tends to reduce the number of hours spent on informal care-giving in the case of long-lasting and severe long-term care needs. This trend requires alternative solutions, including an increase in formal services. As will be shown in chapter 4 in more detail, such an increase in social services can be observed. However, at the same time cost-containment policies nowadays are aimed at strictly limiting institutional care-giving. And even in domiciliary care-giving a concentration on more severely disabled people as well as on nursing and personal help can be observed, whereas domestic and social support are reduced. Herewith, domiciliary care is clearly designed as a complement leaving a considerable amount of care-giving to private, that is mostly informal, solutions. Overall, this tends to create new necessities regarding the possibilities to combine the double burden of work and care.

Similar incentive problems have to be observed with retirement policies (Jackson 1998; Walker, Alber, Guillemard 1993). The well-known issues of financing public pensions in a situation with an increasing number of elderly people, a smaller number of people in the working age population per elderly person, higher life expectancy, increased abilities in later age, etc. have led to policy reforms aimed at increasing retirement age. Welfare policies not only favour this approach because of the cost containment potential in pension policies, but also for productivity reasons.

Apart from the question to what extent there are formal employment opportunities for people in this age-group, the creation of incentives to remain in the labour market means a reduction in the potential of informal work undertaken by people in these age-groups. As shown before, people in their sixties and even later on are important providers of care not only for their grandchildren, but as well for adults in need of long-term care. Men caring for a disabled or a frail elderly person as the main care giver are almost exclusively retired men.

A third example how welfare state policies affect long-term care is income redistribution. Most welfare states not just offer a basic income, but a certain standard of living by relating benefits to income. This – among other consequences – enabled people to live on their own (Prisching 1996). The idea of independent living is strong in modern welfare state ideas. However, solitary living might become a constraint if people do need support in the activities of daily living, for example in moving outdoors or preparing food. 'Economies of scale' realised in co-residence are not possible in the case of solitary living, hence requiring more costly solutions.

Summing up, whereas in most social policy areas the debate about re-organising private and public responsibilities is about shifting responsibilities towards the private sphere (although more the formal than the informal private sphere), the content of the debate in long-term care policies is different. In those countries with traditionally high levels of public support there is a reinforcement of the informal and formal private sphere. In the other countries, recent long-term care policies are very much about introducing public support systems in the community and clarifying the division between private and public responsibilities. As has been shown this may conflict with objectives in other areas of social policy, such as labour market or retirement policies. Furthermore, an overall tendency towards an increasing demand outside informal networks will collide with economic constraints.

Financing the welfare state

All the factors described before – an increasing demand for care, a decreasing ability or willingness to offer long hours of care on a purely informal basis, as well as changes in the social, political and economic environment – tend to require additional resources for long-term care. This has considerably intensified the long-term care debate (see e.g. The Royal Commission on Long Term Care 1999; Wiener 1996; Laing 1993; Davies 1988). Estimations regarding the future costs of long-term care show a considerable increase, even if there is an enormous variation depending on the assumptions regarding the development of disability incidence, the future design of the health and long-term care system and the division between public and private responsibilities (see e.g. Jacobzone, Cambois, Chaplain, Robine 1999; Schmähl, Rothgang 1996; Badelt, Holzmann, Matul, Österle 1996; Laing 1993).

Overall, public expenditure on long-term care as a proportion of total public expenditure and public social expenditure is still comparatively low. (see Table 2.4) For Austria, not included in the study presented in Table 2.4, the respective figure would be about 1% (BMAGS 1999a). Because of considerable variations in definitions and data collecting, figures regarding long-term care expenditure have to be treated with caution. They do however give clear tendencies regarding public involvement in long-term care in Europe. As for the future development of publicly financed long-term care, projections show a substantial increase of long-term care expenditure as a share of GDP. Assuming constant trends for disability rates and institutional settings, it is estimated that this share will increase by about 50% in France and the Netherlands between 2000 and 2020. An even higher increase is estimated for Japan (+ 100%), whereas the increase is lower in Germany (37%), Sweden (+ 27%) or the United Kingdom (+ 20%) (Jacobzone, Cambois, Chaplain, Robine 1999).

Table 2.4 Total social expenditure and public expenditure for long-term care

Country	Social expenditure (% of GDP 1995)	Social expenditure growth [1] (% per year, average 1990-1995)	Public expenditure for long-term care [2] (% of GDP)
Austria	29.7	4.0	n.a.
Belgium	29.7	4.1	0.66
Denmark	34.3	4.5	2.24
Finland	32.8	4.2	0.89
France	30.6	3.1	0.50
Germany	29.4	3.7	0.82
Greece	21.2	n.a.	n.a.
Ireland	19.9	6.1	n.a.
Italy	24.7	1.6	1.00
Luxembourg	25.3	6.8	n.a.
Netherlands	31.4	0.8	1.80
Portugal	20.9	8.7	n.a.
Spain	21.9	3.5	n.a.
Sweden	35.6	n.a.	2.70
United Kingdom	27.7	5.6	1.00

1) Expenditure in purchasing power terms.
2) Estimations by the OECD secretariat for the years 1992 – 1995 (for details see OECD 1998 and Jacobzone 1999).

Source: OECD (1998); European Commission (1998); Jacobzone (1999)

At the same time, public policies and welfare state policies in particular are faced with increased pressures in financing additional benefits. That is, long-term care comes to the top-agenda and tends to require additional resources in an economic situation that is characterised by the objective to stabilise or even reduce public expenditure, and welfare state expenses in particular (Garber 1996).

The reasons for austerity programmes in welfare states are not just to be found in ideological changes and changes in attitudes towards the role of the public and the market sector, or in European Union requirements regarding public expenditure, but in forecasts regarding the dependency ratio. Old-age dependency ratio (to be distinguished from the long-term care dependency ratio discussed before) represents the number of elderly people per person in the working age. Including dependent children gives the total dependency ratio representing the number of dependent people (elderly plus children) per person in the working age. (For a more detailed discussion of various dependency ratios see Jackson 1998.)

Table 2.5 Old-age dependency ratio and total dependency ratio

Country	Old-age dependency ratio [1]			Total dependency ratio [2]		
	1990	2010	2030	1990	2010	2030
Austria	22.4	27.7	44.0	48.2	51.3	71.4
Belgium	22.4	25.6	41.1	49.2	49.3	68.9
Denmark	22.7	24.9	37.7	47.9	51.3	67.0
Finland	19.7	24.3	41.1	48.4	50.4	70.9
France	20.8	24.6	39.1	51.1	51.2	67.9
Germany	21.7	30.3	49.2	45.3	50.0	75.1
Greece	21.2	28.8	40.9	49.6	51.7	66.3
Iceland	16.6	18.1	32.1	55.2	49.5	63.2
Ireland	18.4	18.0	25.3	61.4	51.3	54.5
Italy	21.6	31.2	48.3	45.5	51.5	72.7
Luxembourg	19.9	25.9	44.2	44.8	50.0	72.7
Netherlands	19.1	24.2	45.1	44.5	47.5	73.2
Norway	25.2	24.0	38.7	54.4	51.7	68.3
Portugal	19.5	22.0	33.5	50.7	46.6	59.8
Spain	19.8	23.5	41.0	49.3	46.9	64.8
Sweden	27.6	29.1	39.4	55.3	58.5	70.4
Switzerland	22.0	29.4	48.6	46.1	53.7	77.0
United Kingdom	24.0	25.8	38.7	52.9	52.3	68.0

1) Population aged 65 and over as a percentage of the working age population (15-65 years of age).

2) Population aged 0-14 and 65 and over as a percentage of the working age population (15-65 years of age).

Source: OECD (1996)

According to Table 2.5 the old-age dependency ratio will increase considerably between 1990 and 2010, and even more between 2010 and 2030. Overall, the population aged 65 and over as a proportion of those of a working age will increase from about 20% or slightly above in the year 1990 to about 35% to 45% in the year 2030. Because of decreasing fertility rates, the total dependency ratio tends to show a smaller increase. Downward trends realised by some of the countries in the 1990-2010 period are due to the 'baby-boom' generation entering labour markets. However, overall there tend to be considerably higher burdens on the 'economically active' population.

An expansion of services in long-term care became a public interest at the same time as strict cost-containment policies and the search for increased efficiency came to the top-agenda of social policy. As for cost-containment and efficiency, recent policy approaches in long-term care are characterised by supporting care in the community and by restrictions in institutional care. This includes a reduction of long stays in hospitals as well as a reduction of beds in nursing homes. As for the latter, there is no general reduction in the number of beds – in a number of countries even an increase – but residential care settings nowadays tend to be aimed at those with more severe care needs.

The question of macro-efficiency (Barr 1998), that is the efficient share of means spent for long-term care, collides with an overall situation where total expenditure on welfare is to be held constant (at least as expressed as a policy concern). Consequently, an increase in one sector means a reduction in another sector. This situation supports long-term care solutions that do not just increase public expenditure for long-term care but attempt to balance public and private obligations, which in fact is the direction of a number of recent policy reforms (see part 4).

As can be seen from this discussion of present and future care needs as well as the environment in which care needs have to be dealt with, long-term care issues will require much more attention within social policy in the coming decades. Before looking in more detail at the long-term care system, by investigating the concept and analysing the mix of actors and policies, a clarification of the content and the definition of long-term care is necessary.

2.2 Defining and measuring long-term care

The OECD defines long-term care as 'Any form of care provided consistently over an extended period of time, with no predetermined finishing date, to a person with a long-standing limiting condition or who is at risk of neglect or injury.' (Kalisch, Aman, Buchele 1998)

This definition emphasises two aspects, that is duration (extended period of time and lack of predetermined finishing date) and the characteristics of the person in need of care (a person with a long-standing limiting condition or who is at risk of neglect or injury). Although the definition gives a very good picture of what is meant by long-term care, it still leaves some considerable room for interpretation, especially in the definition of the people in need of care. Broadly speaking long-term care covers frail elderly people as well as disabled people. Here, the term disability will be used for both groups (which is the dominant term in measurement), whereas otherwise the term 'frail elderly' is much more common in discussing long-term care issues, pointing at the majority of people concerned, but neglecting another group.

Long-term care issues are often equated with the elderly population. However, long-term care as defined in this study does not just cover elderly people, but people in all age groups. Disabled children or disabled people in their working age do of course have specific needs or requirements other than those of elderly disabled people. But, as far as long-term care as defined here is concerned, this is not necessarily related with age. This also becomes obvious with focusing just on the elderly population. The dividing line between those in need of long-term care is not a specific age, but the individual situation. Among those in their 60s – although this is an age-group that often is addressed in long-term care policies or long-term care research as the group of potential care receivers – there are more people offering informal long-term care than there are people receiving long-term care.

As for defining and measuring disability and long-term care needs there are at least three concepts that are used: impairments, the inability or the limitations in fulfilling certain activities, and the amount of help needed.

Measurement of *impairments* is concerned with dysfunctions on the physical or mental level, resulting from any cause such as diseases or accidents. This is the dominant measurement approach used in traditional health care, where usually one or at least a small number of such dysfunctions can be identified. Disabled people on the other hand often face multi-morbidity. To what extent this creates the need for support by others, depends on a variety of factors.

Impairments have consequences in terms of *functional performance*. Individuals are restricted in their ability to perform certain activities. Indexes, such as the ADL index ('Activities of Daily Living', e.g. eating, dressing and undressing, moving outdoors, etc.) and the IADL index ('Instrumental Activities of Daily Living', e.g. shopping, taking medicine, handling money, etc.), are used to measure these restrictions. Apart from the fact that there is no standard list of the activities to be covered by such indexes, variation is produced with answer categories in such indexes. A 'yes-no' categorisation might give a quite different picture from a categorisation using three or four levels of restrictions in ADLs and IADLs.

A further distinction is made by WHO (1980) pointing out that the extent of limitations in performing activities not only depends on the individual. In the WHO terminology 'disability' represents disturbances at the individual level, whereas 'handicap' is used for the disadvantages experienced by the individual as a result of impairments and disabilities including the 'design' of the individual's environment. For example, moving outdoors is not only a question of physical restrictions. Mobility also depends on the design of the home, of public transport, or public buildings.

Thirdly, one can look at the amount and/or the frequency of *help and support needed*. Regarding the aim of long-term care – the provision of care – and the above mentioned problems with measuring impairments and restrictions in functional performance, this seems to be a more appropriate approach. However, other measurement problems occur here. Whether measurement is based on professional evaluation, which professionals are measuring (e.g. doctors, nurses or social workers), how measurement procedures are designed, etc. might produce quite different outcomes.

At the policy level one can find all three approaches, often a mix of these three measurement approaches. In addition, definitions on the policy level include a minimum level of care needs to justify public intervention. For example, the German long-term care insurance defines three levels of disability by the frequency in which help is needed in performing certain ADLs and IADLs. In the Austrian long-term care allowance programme, disability is measured within seven levels by a combination of the amount of time needed for care and qualitative aspects. In addition, there are predefined levels for certain impairments.

The 'content' of care becomes quite important for the actual organisation of long-term care systems. Care contains at least four types of help: skilled medical and nursing care, personal care, domestic support, and social support. Skilled medical and nursing care can only be delivered by professionally trained providers, that is doctors and nurses. Personal care (e.g. bathing), domestic support (e.g. shopping, preparing food, cleaning the house) and social support (e.g. in moving outdoors, attending social activities) cover needs of daily living. In good health, these tasks are undertaken by oneself or organised within family or household networks.

Disabled and frail elderly people are unlikely to return to full health and therefore unable to perform at least some of these activities on their own or they do need support in performing these activities. Many of the tasks can be performed without special training which often works as an incentive to support these tasks on an informal basis. This, however, ignores the specific characteristic of 'care'. Care is not just about fulfilling specific tasks, but involves 'emotional caring, in which the person doing the caring is inseparable from the care given.' (Himmelweit 1995: 8) Debating long-term care mainly focuses on visible tasks, whereas emotional aspects, aspects of intimacy and confidentiality, and the burdens rooted inhere for care givers often remain unrecognised.

Another aspect not explicitly stated in the introductory definition is the emphasis on care instead of cure. Delivery and finance of health and social care is often organised along these lines of differentiating cure and care, with a high level of public responsibility in the health sector (cure), and a considerably lower level of public responsibility in the care sector.

This seems to be a rather clear distinction. In reality, however, the distinction of cure and care is far from being clear-cut. And recent trends in pharmacology will probably even further blur the division between cure, rehabilitation, and care. Cure always includes care, and many people in need of long-term care are in need of cure, in order to prevent deterioration in health. One of the consequences – in combination with other factors such as economic incentives – is a considerable number of people in need of long-term care who are cared for in acute hospitals. This, however, does not always correspond with their medical needs that might be served as effectively in another institutional setting or even at their home. This potentially inefficient way to meet the demand for long-term care services is one of the issues underlying certain reform activities in the health and social care sector aimed at improving the effectiveness of the system (see e.g. Saltman, Figueras 1997).

To summarise, the target group of long-term care are people who face a limiting health condition over an extended period of time with no predetermined finishing date. Long-term care is concerned with the consequences of these limiting health conditions, offering nursing care, personal care, domestic and social support. The theoretical analysis of the long-term care system (chapters 2.3 and 2.4 in this section) as well as the conceptualisation of equity interpretations and implications in long-term care (part 3) will follow this basic definition. The empirical analysis in parts 4 and 5 has to deal with a number of restrictions regarding this definition and the availability of corresponding data. Apart from the diversity in attempts to operationalise the basic definition in policy and in research, the outcome of definitions also varies according to the use in practice (see chapter 4.1).

2.3 The long-term care system

Long-term care is about providing and financing care over an extended period of time. It is aimed at those people in need of care, assistance or support in their physical, psychological, health or social life. The informal, the for-profit, the voluntary (non-profit), and the public sector all may act as providers of services and – at least as mediators – of financial means and as financiers of long-term care. The aim of this chapter is to 'unpack' the mix of means and institutional settings in long-term care.

The process of production and consumption of long-term care

The process of social care involves four stages (Goldberg, et al. 1980; Knapp 1984): the identification of problems and difficulties, the process of assessing respective needs, the provision of help, and the effect of the help provided. Adapting this approach for the purpose of this study leads to a model of long-term care as shown in Figure 2.1.

Figure 2.1 The process of long-term care

recognition of long-term care problems → assessment of care needs → production and consumption of care → effects

Source: Adapted from Goldberg, et al. (1980) and Knapp (1984)

At the beginning of the long-term care 'process' is the occurrence of presumably long-lasting difficulties of individuals in their health status and in their ability to perform certain activities. The recognition of such difficulties is the first impulse to respond to these problems. Recognition might take place in the private informal environment as well as in formal settings, for example in a hospital as a consequence of an acute health problem. With any response to health problems we enter the sphere of 'producing' care. The production of care is about the provision and the finance of care, which are closely interrelated and will be discussed in more detail below. This stage includes the assessment of needs, a process of referral, the actual delivery of help as well as the financing of care.

Before entering the sphere of production and consumption, there are two concepts to be distinguished as a response to the recognition of limitations or restrictions, that is the concept of needs and the specific economic concept of demand. Behind these concepts there are very different ideas about the individual and society and, hence, they are at the core of welfare, welfare societies and welfare states.

Demand exists if there is '... a want for some good or service backed by a willingness to sacrifice resources for it.' (Culyer 1980: 70) According to this concept, the number of people who will demand care depends upon their financial resources and their preferences as well as the relative cost of care. The individual is regarded as the best authority in determining which goods and how these goods are produced and distributed. Economic theory suggests that by following the individuals' self-interest social welfare will be maximised. However, as health and social care, the production of care and the outcome of this production are characterised by a number of particular features – which will be discussed in more detail in this and the following chapter – the demand concept and its relevance to the health and social care sector has attracted a lot of discussion and is confronted with various objections (see e.g. Grossman 1972; Williams 1997).

Need, on the other hand, seems to be an elusive and rather contested concept (Langan 1998; Doyal, Gough 1991) with a broad range of interpretations in the social sciences. Bradshaw (1972) identifies normative need, felt need, expressed need and comparative need. Here, 'normative' need is what an expert or professional defines as need. In long-term care, a medical doctor or a nurse might be such an expert to qualify a situation with regard to the existence of need. 'Felt' and 'expressed' need in this conceptualisation are a response by individuals, either in assessing need by themselves ('felt' need) or in turning this need into action, for example by visiting a doctor or by being put on a waiting list ('expressed' need). 'Comparative' need, finally, exists if an individual does not receive a service, other individuals, however, with similar characteristics do receive that service.

The concept of need is characterised by a range of properties (Kolm 1996; Doyal, Gough 1991). Most important for this study are objective vs. subjective concepts, and herewith the authority to decide on the existence of needs, as well as the nature of needs. Whereas subjective concepts refer to the authority of individuals, either the person in need of care or an external agent or expert, objective concepts believe in universal basic needs. Whereas the neo-classical approach in economics rejects such objective needs, a strong argument for their existence is developed by Doyal, Gough (1991). Among other factors they include physical health and autonomy with a number of intermediate needs, such as physical security or appropriate health care promoting health and autonomy. However, for needs other than purely physical and physiological needs, culture-determined tastes, social relations or norms will play an important role. Hence, for these needs Kolm (1996: 324) follows: 'As a consequence an objective (acultural) definition of an objective need is usually impossible, but the sociological determination of such a need is usually rather clear, and its political revelation is commonly easy and available. Contrary to many others, this problem is difficult (impossible) in theory but easy in practice. Indeed at a moment in time and in a given culture, there typically is a rough consensus about what the important or basic needs are.'

The role given to different concepts of need or the more specific concept of demand in the design of long-term care systems, and herewith the role of the various actors in the field, is – among other determinants – a consequence of specific characteristics of the production of care and at the same time determines the production of care.

There are several aspects that make the production of care different from traditional features of production. It is not just social care that is needed, but better health, improved well-being, or support and assistance because of limitations in specific abilities. Clients are not just consumers of care but involved in the process of producing care. Finally, there are difficulties in defining and assessing the output of the production of care. The social service production function (Culyer 1980), the production of welfare approach (Knapp 1984; Davies, Knapp 1981) and the social production of welfare approach (Netten, Davies 1990) have tried to consider these characteristics in an extended model of production.

The 'social service production function' emphasises the role of clients. It is a key characteristic of personal services that clients have to participate in the production. A specific service, such as meals-on-wheels, is not the final focus of care but a means to achieve a final outcome. In the process of producing a final outcome the client is not just the receiver of an outcome but becomes an actor in the production process (Culyer 1980).

The recognition of different stages in the production of health or well-being is a major challenge in health economics. (For an introduction see e.g. Folland, Goodman, Stano 1997 or Zweifel, Breyer 1997.) Here, a distinction is made between production functions focusing on the *production of health care* and those focusing on the *production of health*. In the latter case, health as the dependent variable is measured by mortality rates, morbidity rates, disability days or a variety of quality-of-life measures. Health care is regarded as just one among a number of factors that determine health. Other variables include economic factors, such as income, organisational factors, such as physician density or information, life style factors or education. Studies are pointing out that many of these factors other than the actual health care production are most important as determinants for health outcome (see e.g. Fuchs 1974; Wolfe 1986). Whereas the overall importance of variables outside the health care sector is without doubt, there is mixed evidence for the direction and strength of causality between variables and the reasons for the relationships observed.

The same idea of stages in the production is to be found in the 'production of welfare' approach where a distinction is made between intermediate outputs and final outputs (Knapp 1984). In this approach services provided, such as meals-on-wheels or home help services, are defined as intermediate outputs. The final output is changes in the health and well-being status of the clients, in the case of meals-on-wheels – technically speaking – satisfaction in the need for nutrition. The main argument of the production of welfare approach is that, given exactly the same kind of meal, the level of satisfaction might differ quite considerably.

This argument is related to another specific property of social care. The final output not only depends on the quantity and quality of the intermediate output, but on additional factors, such as attitudes and experiences in the care environment or clients' characteristics. In the production of welfare approach these are called non-resource inputs as they are neither physical nor tangible. Although the role of clients and the wider quality of care is central to social work approaches, these non-resource inputs tend to be underestimated or even ignored in the analysis of long-term care issues. This is also because of problems in assessing the relevance of these characteristics. For example: A lower level in the number of beds in residential care settings per 1,000 elderly people in country A compared to another country B represents differences in the intermediate output, but does not necessarily mean that the final outcome is smaller in country A with a lower number of beds per 1,000 elderly people. Apart from the availability of alternative care settings, preferences regarding the type of care-giving might differ quite considerable between countries.

It has already been shown (chapter 2.1) that informal care-giving plays a key role in the production of long-term care. This, however, has been widely neglected in research and policy analysis and only recently there is an increasing recognition of this input. The informal sector might be – and in fact to a considerable extent is – involved in all the stages described before: the recognition of the problem, the assessment of needs, and the provision as well as the finance of long-term care. What makes the analysis more difficult is not just the fact that these actors are outside the formal sector, but also because there is an unclear division of responsibilities between the formal and the informal sector and again the question of measuring and valuing this item.

Figure 2.2 An extended model of the production and consumption of long-term care

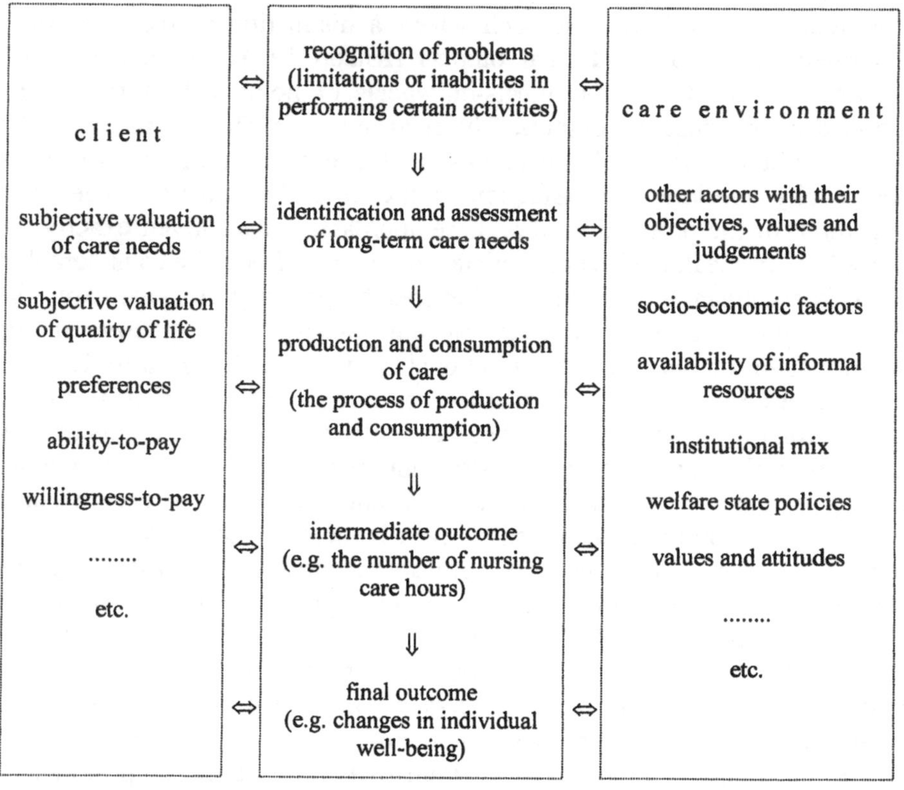

The 'social production of welfare' approach (Netten, Davies 1990) offers a theoretical framework to recognise and to integrate informal networks. The model, based on the 'new home economics' (see e.g. Quah 1993), extends the basic unit of production and consumption from the household to the informal care network which is seen as the basic unit of the production of welfare.

Including these considerations in the process shown in Figure 2.1 leads to an extended model as described in Figure 2.2, which explicitly recognises the central role of those in need of care as well as the 'care environment' in all the stages of the process of care. The actual production of nursing care, personal care, domestic and social support contains the provision and the finance of care and will be looked at in more detail below, analysing the mix of means and institutional settings in these spheres.

The institutional mix in long-term care

The institutional mix is the different types of organisational forms to be found as actors in a specific policy field. In economics, this is very much dually dominated by the private (for-profit) and the public sector. But long-term care is a prime example where these two organisational forms just reflect part of the whole picture with a comparatively small role for the for-profit market sector. At least four different settings have to be distinguished: the informal sector, the private for-profit sector, the non-profit sector, and the public sector (Evers, Olk 1996; Evers, Svetlik 1993).

In a (perfectly functioning) for-profit market, resources are allocated according to consumers' preferences, ability and willingness to pay. The market is accessible to those who are able and willing to pay for long-term care. The potential role of the market in long-term care includes benefits for employees, the provision of commercially produced goods as residential care settings and social services or private long-term care insurance solutions. Overall, evidence shows a comparatively small role of for-profit market solutions in long-term care. Some arguments, mainly from the economics literature, why this might be the case are presented in chapter 2.4. Beyond these efficiency and allocational concerns the distributional outcome of pure market solutions might not be seen as desirable.

The private non-profit sector is characterised by considerable variations in formality and professionalism. Despite heterogeneity, all models are oriented at specific needs to be satisfied without taking the individuals' ability-to-pay as a major criterion in the allocation of resources. The role of the non-profit sector might be a complement or a substitute to other sectors. Although the non-profit sector often has been seen as the sector stepping in where other sectors fail, it might as well be the other sectors fulfilling this role. Overall, the diversity of the non-profit sector contains potential as well as problems for these organisations (see e.g. Badelt 1999). With regard to long-term care, non-profit organisations are important providers in the residential as well as in the domiciliary care sector (see part 4). They are not in a position to offer social welfare as rights, they may, however, play an important role as lobbies or as agents for those with specific needs.

In the state sector resources are allocated according to legal rights, although there might be considerable room for discretionary decisions on the various bureaucratic levels. The role of the state in long-term care includes regulation as well as – potentially – finance, purchasing and provision. Only recently, the role of the state to supplement and to relief the informal care-giving sector is slightly more recognised by approaching carers not just as resources but also as clients. The state sector has strong potential for guaranteeing equal access to services across a country. It might, however, also neglect specific needs or reduce the potential role of other institutional sectors. Choices made by the state sector in long-term care with regard to equity objectives will be discussed in depth in part 5.

Last but certainly not least in long-term care, the informal sector is that of primary relationships, of families and households – which are most important in long-term care – as well as neighbours and friends. The allocation of resources among members of the smaller community follows aspects such as altruism, reciprocity, or mutual respect. In long-term care, informal care-giving still makes the bulk of care-giving (see chapter 2.1) offering care or financial support to dependent members of the family or the small social community. Those, however, who are not member of such a smaller community do not have access to this kind of care-giving. Given increasing financial pressure to provide publicly financed services, quality assurance became a major issue in all the institutional settings in order to prevent deterioration of quality or to improve the quality of care. Consequently, carers in the informal sector are increasingly seen in their different roles, as resources, as co-workers and as co-clients (Twigg 1990). Respective policy measures, however, are in most countries only at the beginning (see part 4).

These four types are just the basic models in the institutional mix. In a real world perspective, various mixed forms are to be identified. Boundaries between the four sectors are vague and will probably become even more so. In the public sector, apart from actors on the federal, the local and the community level, parafiscal or quasi-governmental organisations act as purchasers or providers. Contracting-out services or public-private partnerships represent shared responsibilities between the public and the private (either for-profit or non-profit) sector. Payments for care or social security arrangements for informal carers are aimed at reducing the 'informality' of that sector. Within the non-profit sector there are those organisations acting as almost quasi-public sector organisations if they are fully funded by the public sector and organisationally closely linked. Others have strong links to the community emphasising voluntary work, participation or self-help.

The design of the institutional mix ('welfare mix', 'welfare pluralism') is one of the characteristic features of recent developments in social policy and receives increasing attention as a specific approach in social policy research (e.g. Evers, Olk 1996; Wistow, Knapp, Hardy, Allen 1993). Regarding the institutional mix in long-term care, it is estimated that in the European Union countries more than two thirds of care is provided in the informal sector, whereas 13% is public service, 11% privately paid services and 3% services from volunteers (Walker 1995). However, there are enormous differences in the actual design of the various systems with regard to the extent of the four sectors as well as the role of and relations between the sectors (see part 4). Overall, the mix of institutional settings to be found in long-term care systems makes it a prime example for the welfare mix approach.

The provision of long-term care

Long-term care is about fulfilling needs – arising from limiting conditions in the individual's state of health – over an extended period of time. Long-term care needs include the need for skilled medical and nursing care, personal care, domestic support as well as social support and might be covered by in-kind services or – on an intermediate stage – payments enabling recipients to pay for services.

The in-kind response to long-term care needs – if recognised as such – includes the delivery of health and social care services either in the home of the client or in a specific environment outside the home of the client with an increasing diversification in services (see e.g. Pacolet, Bouten, Lanoye, Versieck 2000; Kane 1995). In the latter case services might be provided in an environment which the client enters just for receiving specific services (e.g. a day centre or a social services centre) or in an environment which becomes the living environment for the client (e.g. a nursing home, a residential home or – for a limited period of time – even a hospital). As shown in a number of studies (e.g. Portrait, Lindeboom, Deeg 2000; Klein 1996; Rhoades 1998; Schulz-Nieswandt 1994; Shapiro, Tate 1988), institutionalisation not only depends on the severity of chronic illnesses and the extent of care needs, but also on issues such as marital status, the walking distance to public transport, and incentives to be found in the overall organisation of the long-term care system. Most studies reveal that factors other than the health status and related needs become more important with better health.

Regarding cost-effectiveness, care at home is generally seen as favourable compared to care in residential care settings, at least up to a certain amount of care needs. This result, however, is restricted by problems in the identification and measurement of a number of input as well as outcome variables (e.g. Badelt, Holzmann, Matul, Österle 1996; Davies, Knapp 1981). Observed advantages in terms of cost-effectiveness arise from at least the following two facts: First, services in the community tend to support clients only where clients would otherwise be limited in the performance of certain activities, whereas in residential care settings an extended amount of support is offered (e.g. with the preparation of meals for all the residents). Second, care in the community always includes informal support which is rather limited in residential care settings. Problems in measuring informal care often lead to a neglect of informal care in quantitative analyses and, hence, to an overestimation of the advantages of care in the community regarding cost-effectiveness. Hence, a recognition of informal inputs in the long-term care production in the form of opportunity costs might have considerable consequences for the abovementioned advantages of community care with regard to cost-effectiveness (Carmichael, Charles 1998; Ettner 1996). On the other hand, it is argued that the expansion of social services will not reduce total expenditure. This is because the majority of those receiving social services would remain in their home even if social services would not be available and because the effect of an increase in social services on an extension of those people consuming such services is stronger than the effect of reducing the number of people living in residential care settings (Kemper, Applebaum, Harrigan 1987; Leutz 1986).

A further impact on cost-effectiveness of community vs. residential care arises from the quality of care. Here, the challenges for the evaluation arises from considerable problems in the identification and measurement of the output or outcome of care and hence quality. As will be shown this might be an obstacle to individual judgements by disabled or frail elderly people as well as to evaluations by experts or professionals (see chapter 2.4).

Apart from in-kind provision in various settings, provision might also be initiated by cash payments which then can be used to organise necessary care. Cash benefits as a substitute or as a complement to services recently became more prominent on the long-term care agenda shifting purchasing power to receivers of such payments. Payments for care evolve in a wide range of forms. Payments might be directed to care receivers or to carers in the informal or voluntary sector. They may take the form of direct or indirect payments. Direct payments include payments related to the work provided, related to foregone wages or related to contributions paid. Indirect payments include tax credits or tax reductions, financial support for specific care-related expenditure, as well as – in the case of payments to carers – the recognition of care work for social security rights (Pijl 1994). Regarding problems in the 'final targeting' of cash payments, some propose vouchers as an alternative to cash (e.g. Nocera, Zweifel 1996). Paying carers – be it carers within family networks or volunteers – raises a number of questions with regard to, e.g., a blurring dichotomy between regular employment and informal care, paid and unpaid work, paid volunteering, etc. And – depending on the actual design – it might conflict heavily with other welfare state issues such as labour market or gender equality concerns (Ungerson 2000; Ungerson 1997; Ungerson 1995; Evers 1994; Glendinning, McLaughlin 1993; Baldock, Ungerson 1991; Leat 1990).

Care-giving covers a broad range of tasks requiring different levels of training and experience. Many tasks involve close emotional relationships to the person providing the actual care. Regarding the organisation of long-term care, this has important implications for the institutional mix in the provision of care and the division between the formal and the informal sector. Different options regarding actors and policies in the provision of long-term care are shown in Table 2.6. Families, other informal networks (including the wider family network, neighbours, friends and volunteers), non-profit organisations, for-profit organisations, and the public sector all may act as providers of long-term care. Means of support in long-term care are in-kind provision (including social and health services in the community, residential care settings, a number of mixed types such as day care centres as well as informal care), cash benefits from the welfare state as well as from private sources (enabling recipients to pay for care) and the regulation of provision. As will be shown in part 4, the mix of institutional alternatives, the borderline between public and private responsibilities as well as the mix of what is actually provided varies considerably between and even within countries.

Even in systems with a relatively high level of social service support, the bulk of care-giving is offered by informal providers, i.e. household and family members and – of minor importance – friends and neighbours. Apart from the dominant form of informal care-giving as in-kind provision, private transfers also occur, in particular from family members outside the care receivers' household. As for the actual provision in the informal sector, there usually is one main care giver who, most of the time, is a woman. Male care givers in general are retired whereas many women have to either combine work in the formal sector and care in the informal sector or – at least partly – to withdraw from formal employment (e.g. Jani-Le Bris 1993; Glendinning, McLaughlin 1993; Hoskins 1993; Badelt, Holzmann-Jenkins, Matul, Österle 1997).

Tablc 2.6 Resources in the provision of long-term care

Providers	*cash payments as intermediate means*	*in-kind provision*
Families Other informal networks	private transfers	informal care-giving
Non-profit organisations	(insurance payments)	social services residential care
For-profit organisations	(insurance payments)	social services residential care
Social insurance Public sector	tax-based payments insurance payments regulating payments	social services residential care regulating provision

(...) indicates that this mode of finance is of no or very limited practical relevance

Although long-term care was always overwhelmingly delivered in the informal sector, informal long-term care-giving has been widely ignored in the design and in the analysis of long-term care policies. Only with increasing awareness of the problems associated with long-term informal care-giving, the risk of loosing a considerable amount of this 'hidden' resource and increasing financial pressures, informal care receives more attention. In this study informal care-giving and the equity implications of long-term care policies on informal care givers will be discussed in the context of financing long-term care (see below).

In-kind provision and cash payments are to be found in the formal and informal private as well as in the public sector. Apart from the historical development of long-term care systems and the cultural and socio-economic background, the role of the various actors depends on the purchasing power in the hands of care receivers, the recognition of long-term care as a (social) risk, whether long-term care is regarded as a welfare state issue and how and to what extent public intervention occurs. Regarding the division between the formal and the informal sector, there is an increase in the use of services in both sectors when someone is more severely disabled, however the increase tends to be even stronger in the informal sector. In addition, the use of formal care tends to increase with income (e.g. Kemper 1992; Coughlin, McBride, Perozek, Liu 1992). Regarding those cohorts in the population who are most at risk to need long-term care in the future, this might lead to an even bigger increase in the demand for formal care provision than it would be caused by the socio-demographic developments discussed in chapter 2.1.

The formal private sector is represented by the for-profit and the non-profit sector, with the non-profit sector clearly dominating the for-profit sector in most countries. Although the specific risk structure could make long-term care a case for a private insurance solution, the establishment or the expansion of for-profit initiatives is rather limited even in countries where public support is restricted to means-tested social assistance (Hennessy, 1997; Garber, 1996; Wiener 1998). The reason for the rather small role of the for-profit sector can be found in a number of market failure issues that will be briefly discussed in chapter 2.4. (For a more detailed discussion in long-term care see e.g. Sievering 1996; Felder, Zweifel 1998; Davis, Rowland 1986.) Pauly (1990) searching for other reasons for the very limited role of the private for-profit sector argues that nonpurchase of long-term care insurance is rational when family members represent an alternative source of care, because the main consequence of coverage than would be an enhancement of the expected value of one's estate.

The non-profit sector is a very heterogeneous sector. It ranges from non-profit organisations working without volunteers, to non-profit organisations combining paid and voluntary employment, to actors organising help by volunteers or neighbours setting up some sort of co-operative initiative. The role of non-profit organisations in the long-term care system ranges from charities depending on a wide range of financial sources to partners in contracting-out models, where purchase and actual provision is divided between the public and the formal private sector, and from the primary supplier in the formal sector in some countries to a subsidiary supplier role in other countries.

The role of the public sector in providing long-term care and regulating provision is characterised by shared responsibilities between different levels of public bodies. Apart from giving a general direction in policies, the role of central public bodies often is rather restricted compared to local public bodies. However, there is and there will probably continue to be an increasingly important role in imposing general directions and setting quality standards in order to reduce inequalities in service provision within countries. This often is, but does not have to be connected with the finance of care. Central governments also play an important role if social insurance solutions and payment for care programmes are established, which tend to be more standardised within countries than social services. The actual provision of services by public bodies is usually dominated by those on a local level. Here, the establishment of residential care settings has often been seen as the adequate public response, an approach which today is regarded as highly inefficient and inequitable. A redefinition of the role of the state in welfare provision in many countries has lead to a purchaser and provider split, that is the public sector acts as a financier of long-term care provision whereas the actual delivery of services is formally contracted-out to providers in the for-profit or the non-profit market sector. In the case of payments for care, control of the public sector over the form and the extent of service provision is further reduced.

The role of the public sector as a regulatory body is on the central as well as on local levels. Regulating the provision of long-term care includes a wide range of issues, such as the allocation of responsibilities in the provision of care among various actors, the regulation of eligibility criteria and access for those in need of care; regulations might include standards regarding the qualification and training of professional providers, standards for the actual provision of care, etc. More recent trends to split the role of purchaser and provider, to contract out services, to increase diversification in the institutional mix as well as the growing importance of quality and accountability might strengthen the regulatory role on the central as well as on local levels.

The finance of long-term care

Long-term care is not just about the mode and the extent of care provided, but also about who is paying for care. In the light of an estimated considerable increase in the need for care (see chapter 2.1), discussions on the finance of long-term care have intensified in recent years (see e.g. Amaradio 1998; Parker, Clarke 1997; Laing 1993; Davies 1988). These discussions are heavily concentrated on the formal sector. Proposals for reforms vary considerably according to the weight that is given to the basic objectives of efficiency and equity (see e.g. The Royal Commission on Long-Term Care 1999; Scanlon 1992; Laing 1993; Schmähl 1992; Eisen 1992). The role of the informal sector is usually discussed separately, completely ignored or just briefly touched upon in many of the general discussions about how to organise the finance of long-term care. This study attempts to bring the issues together by analysing equity implications in the finance of care including informal care as a mode of in-kind financing.

Paying for welfare is characterised by mixed modes of finance (Glennerster 1997). In the finance of long-term care – as with the provision of care – contributions in cash and contributions in kind can be distinguished as the main ways of financing care. Contributions in cash include cash payments, either out-of-pocket, from savings or assets, private insurance contributions, social insurance contributions, and taxes. Informal and voluntary care-giving, or in fact the time spent on informal care-giving, is the in-kind input most relevant. Other in-kind inputs are more of a conceptual interest than because of their practical relevance.

Cash payments play an important role in long-term care. They may be used to pay for services in the formal as well as in the informal sector. In the informal sector payments are either made to informal carers, to volunteers or to care providers in a grey economy. Whereas the role of market solutions with full coverage by clients is rather limited, co-payments for services received from suppliers in the formal private and the public sector do play an increasing role. Co-payments evolve in different forms: payments that cover specific kinds of services (e.g. the hotel component in nursing homes), flat-rate payments, means-tested co-payments, etc. The individual source of these payments are income and savings. In the case of long-lasting and severe health limitations costs will exceed regular income of most individuals. If there is neither extensive informal care available nor broad coverage by public services or benefits, most people will have to use their savings (and sometimes that of close family members) to make the necessary payments. As will be shown in section four, many countries are searching for a middle approach, including co-payments by clients but at the same time attempting to prevent considerable drops in the living standard because of long-lasting care needs.

The other forms of financing long-term care through cash payments are to be found in the formal sector. It has already been mentioned that the purchase of private insurance – and herewith the role of private insurance contributions – is rather limited. For the United States it is estimated that only about 4% to 5% of elderly people do have private insurance coverage for long-term care needs and just 1% of residential care costs are paid out of private insurance (Wiener, Illston, Hanley 1994). Figures for Europe are even lower (Pacolet, Bouten, Lanoye, Versieck 1999b). The future possibilities of a system of private insurance that does not take account of different income situations seems restricted as it is estimated that just a rather small proportion of the population could afford such an insurance. For example, the estimated share of those in the United States for whom private long-term care insurance would be affordable is no more than 20%

(Binstock 1998). Going beyond this share would require significant regulatory and financial public intervention (Wiener 1998).

As far as the public sector as long-term care financier is concerned, financial sources are based on social insurance contributions and taxes. Whereas social insurance contributions tend to be earmarked, this is the exception with taxes. Earmarking with taxes may, however, occur if long-term care is partly financed through tax reductions or tax exemptions related to long-term care needs as proposed by the Clinton administration in the United States (The New York Times - January 4, 1999). All the existing forms of public finance are far from covering all care needs (Scanlon 1992). Even specific care needs, such as nursing care, often require co-payments.

Apart from cash contributions, financing long-term care may be based on in-kind contributions. In-kind contributions in the formal sector – e.g. in-kind transfers in a co-operative organisation or compulsory social service – are not at all widespread. In-kind contributions in the informal sector, however, are the main source of financing long-term care.

Long-term care-giving is a scarce resource as any other economic good whose usage creates considerable opportunity costs. A number of studies dealing with these questions demonstrate and evaluate the opportunity costs of informal long-term care. Informal care-giving tasks tend to be most burdensome, physically and emotionally. Many carers face a considerable amount of total work hours per week, whether they combine formal employment and informal care-giving or they have to provide long hours of care. On what terms formal employment and informal care-giving have to be combined is another source of opportunity costs. Withdrawal from as well as reducing formal employment to part-time work has negative consequences in terms of employment, career opportunities, income status, as well as the position in the social security system (e.g. Carmichael, Charles 1998; Ettner 1996; Holzmann, Österle 1996; Phillips 1994; Glendinning 1992).

Recent policy initiatives such as payment for care programmes or the introduction of social insurance coverage for informal care givers are a first step to increasingly interfere in this domain. The broader implications of such approaches on the social and economic situation of informal care givers, however, are rather controversial (see above).

Despite the fact that informal care without direct compensation is the main source of financing long-term care, informal long-term care-giving tends to be either ignored or addressed in studies specifically aimed at the issue of informal care. Any neglect of the value of the informal sector in the analysis of efficiency or equity issues in long-term care leads to considerably distorted results. Although problems with defining and measuring the value of informal long-term care might cause severe variations and probably make quantitative analysis inadequate for specific questions, implications should at least be discussed in qualitative terms whenever efficiency or equity of long-term care systems is investigated.

Combining modes of paying for care and institutional alternatives, five basic models for the finance of care can be identified (Table 2.7): two party models (care receiver and care giver) and three different third party models, where a third party is involved as a financier of care.

Table 2.7 Burdens in the finance of long-term care

Finance	*Contributions*	
	in cash	*in kind*
Informal two party model (care receiver + care giver)	cash payments (using pocket money, savings, assets)	time spent on informal care-giving
Formal two party model (care receiver + care giver)	cash payments (using pocket money, savings, assets)	(in-kind transfers in a co-operative system)
Informal third party model (care receiver + care giver + informal networks)	cash transfers	in-kind transfers
Private third party model (care receiver + care giver + private insurance)	private insurance contributions	(in-kind transfers in a co-operative system)
Public third party model (care receiver + care giver + public sector / social insurance)	taxes social insurance contributions regulating finance	(compulsory in-kind transfers) regulating finance

(...) indicates that this mode of finance is of no or very limited practical relevance.

In the two party models, care receivers either make out-of-pocket payments to buy care, or care is offered on an informal basis as an in-kind contribution without direct compensation. The latter is the dominant form in purely private informal care relationships, leaving (non)remuneration of these burdens to internal family or household processes. In the case of cash payments the two party model might take different forms: In the informal sector model, parties are part of a smaller social community such as the family, household or a network of friends and neighbours. In the formal private sector model payments are made for the actual care-giving. There are, however, vague boundaries between the informal and the formal sector. On the one hand, volunteering plays a substantial role in long-term care and payment for care programmes tend to promote an expansion and diversification of the various models of volunteering (Evers 1994). On the other hand, payments for care create incentives for a grey economy becoming increasingly widespread in some countries' long-term care systems (see e.g. Gori 2001). Here, the relationship is not formal in the sense that it is based on regular employment contracts or regular organisational settings, but at the same time it is not informal in the sense that it is based on family or other close personal relationships (Göke, Hartwig 1998; Ungerson 1995; Evers 1994).

In the third party models additional actors enter the care arena. In the informal third party model individuals act as informal financiers of long-term care. This might be family members apart from the main care giver, friends or neighbours offering care, or family members transferring money to the person in need of care or to the main care giver enabling them to buy specific aids or care services.

Though there are some characteristics that would make long-term care a case for risk management via private insurance, such formal private third party models are rather limited as has been shown above. Without public intervention problems in establishing private insurance contracts occur even in countries were the role of the public sector is rather limited. In-kind transfers in the private third party model represent the idea of co-operatives according to the insurance idea, where services are offered as contributions instead of cash contributions. Apart from grass-root initiatives, this has almost no importance for the design of long-term care systems.

Restrictions in financing long-term care out of income or savings in the case of long-lasting care needs and problems with purely private third party models have lead to the evolution of a wide range of public third party models. Yet, the existing models are far less developed than, for example, those in health care or public pension systems. Whereas the finance of long-term care through tax or social insurance systems is mostly organised on the central level, the specific use of funds may well be decentralised. A form of in-kind contribution – of little importance in the real design of long-term care systems – are compulsory in-kind transfers. However, through regulations the public sector obliges family members in a number of countries to contribute to the finance of long-term care through in-kind or cash contributions. Apart from regulations touching upon the informal sector, public bodies tend to have an increasing role in regulating the formal private sector if private insurance or compulsory private insurance solutions are favoured. Hence, the public sector increasingly intervenes in the allocation of responsibilities in the formal and in the informal sphere of financing care.

The design of long-term care systems is characterised by a combination of formal and informal structures, and a public-private mix that recognises social responsibilities alongside individual responsibility. Apart from the institutional mix, long-term care systems are characterised by a broad range of modes of delivering and financing long-term care. As will be shown in more detail in part 4 of this study, this mix of the aforementioned policy approaches regarding means and institutional settings does not only reflect potential elements in the design of a long-term care system, but can be found in a wide range even within single countries. This makes the institutional and policy mix a major characteristic of long-term care systems.

2.4 Long-term care as a welfare state issue

This study attempts to explore the role of the welfare state in the establishment of an equitable allocation of resources and burdens in long-term care through choices in the design of the provision and finance of long-term care. The broad range of potential institutional settings in which long-term care can be organised raises a number of questions regarding the institutional mix and the issues that might make long-term care a welfare state concern. According to the economics of the welfare state (e.g. Barr 1998) and the public choice literature (e.g. Mueller 1989), the existence and the extent of state activity can be explained within different sets of reasons:

- state intervention for reasons of allocational market failure
- welfare as a merit good
- state intervention for distributional concerns
- the role of governments, the electorate, pressure groups, and bureaucrats

In the case of allocational *market failure*, state intervention is argued for based on assumptions of efficient allocation via private markets that do not hold. Economic theory has widely analysed the arguments of natural monopoly, public goods, externalities, and imperfect information, some of which might cause market failure in long-term care which in turn might be used as a justification for state intervention in the allocation of scarce resources in long-term care.

As has been shown in a number of studies, the natural monopoly situation – that is increasing returns to scale at all relevant levels of output – does not occur in long-term care (e.g. McKay 1988; Kass 1987). The same is true for public goods, characterised by two features, according to which a) it is impossible to exclude a person from the benefits if this person has not paid specifically for this benefit, and b) there is no rivalry between beneficiaries. External effects and information problems, however, might cause inefficiency in purely private long-term care market solutions.

External effects are realised when an economic transaction effects a third party without being involved in the transaction. Different aspects have to be considered for long-term care (e.g. Bradley 1998; Sievering 1996; Culyer 1980). Positive externalities might be borne by family members as well as the larger society. On the one hand, positive externalities are produced if family members and/or the larger community do not have to provide long-term care if a long-term care insurance is purchased by the individual. As private long-term care insurance is still the exception, there might be caring externalities, which are of particular importance for long-term care. Caring externalities (or psychological externalities) are characterised by interdependent utility functions that are not only determined by the individual consumption, but by the consumption of others. That is, the consumption of care has positive effects on others, in particular on close family members but on the larger community as well. If such caring externalities exist, the amount of care provided by pure market solutions derived from individuals' self-interest will be smaller than in a solution recognising these externalities.

As a fourth argument informational problems are put forward, which are in fact often seen as the major argument for market failure in long-term care (Bradley 1998; Sievering 1996). Long-term care needs do not necessarily occur in one's lifetime. However, if long-term care needs occur, costs tend to be considerable and will exceed the ability-to-pay of many individuals in need of care. Because of the specific risk-structure, individual risk-management leading to private insurance schemes would be expected. But, even in countries where public support for long-term care is limited to social assistance, the importance of private insurance is either small or almost negligible. The main reasons for this effect are sought in information problems. Others argue that nonpurchase of long-term care insurance might be rational if family members as an alternative source of care and preferences regarding bequests are taken into account (Pauly 1990).

There are several types of information problems that might occur in long-term care: moral hazard, adverse selection, imperfect information on alternative schemes in the provision and finance of care, as well as imperfect information on the quality of care (see e.g. Bradley 1998; Sievering 1990). Moral hazard means that individuals reduce their efforts to prevent the need for long-term care because the risk is covered by insurance or by any other external funds. Additionally, there is more room for supply-side induced demand if contributions of the individuals in need of care are not related to what they actually consume. Obviously, moral hazard is not just a problem of the private market solution, but might also occur in compulsory insurance or tax financed schemes. But the consequences might be different. Moral hazard requires higher insurance premiums. In this case, in the private sector individuals will tend to quit the insurance contract leaving them in a situation where the risk is covered by individual income, wealth and finally social assistance. In compulsory insurance solutions, higher premiums might be accepted to some extent in order to guarantee distributional objectives. But there are approaches to reduce moral hazard – for example by introducing control mechanisms or co-payments – in both models.

Adverse selection might occur in two ways. If those (potentially) in need of care are better informed about their health status, there will be a tendency of bad risks to be covered by insurance leading again to higher premiums, whereas the 'good risks' will search for other solutions. On the other hand, 'cream-skimming' might occur if insurers are able to select good risks. In both cases, compulsory insurance could reduce negative distributional effects, however, for the price of increased moral hazard.

Imperfect information may also lead to deficiencies in choosing among alternative financing or provision schemes (Bradley 1998). As suggested by behavioural studies, improving information is not just about improving the availability and dissemination of information, for example, by reducing the social isolation of many people in need of long-term care. Decision-making in long-term care is also characterised by the individual's disabilities or limitations that might reduce the ability to search, use and process information. In addition, there is the complexity of actors that might be involved in the decision-making process. Apart from the individual in need of care, these are members of the family or other personal networks, experts and professionals such as doctors, nurses, home helpers or bureaucrats.

Finally, information problems occur in the context of measuring and monitoring the quality of care (see e.g. Nocon, Qureshi 1996). This aspect has already been touched upon when discussing the production of care vs.

the production of a final output. The intermediate outcome or – in economic terminology – output is the actual delivery and receipt of services such as the number of visits from the home nurse or the time spent by a home help service with the care receiver. The final outcome or output is the effect or impact on the service user, that is the person in need of care. Problems in identifying and measuring this final outcome makes it critical for individual decision-making – and, hence, the efficient allocation of resources in a private market system – as well as in any decision-making process involving additional actors. The number of hours spent by home help services does not necessarily give an indication of the effectiveness of this service and the number of residential care settings per 1,000 elderly people does not necessarily indicate whether this is appropriate for the individuals living in the respective area.

Different aspects of this kind of information problems have to be distinguished. First of all, the objectives in long-term care, and hence the relevant aspects of the outcome, might differ quite considerably. On the one hand, they differ between various domains, e.g. physical well-being, emotional well-being, social integration. Frail elderly people with identical physical limitations might have very different ideas about their needs. This would suggest the demand concept as the optimal approach to satisfy these needs. However, as discussed before, the demand concept tends to be restricted in health and social care. The complexity of the decision-making process includes other actors, whose objectives might differ from those people in need of care. The necessity and appropriateness of being cared for in a residential care setting, for example, might be seen quite different from the person in need of care, close family members or experts responsible for the assessment of care needs. If the various aspects of the outcome are identified, further problems arise with measuring outcome and, hence, the quality of care and the quality of the outcome, altogether a most difficult task or the gordian knot in long-term care (Gibson 1998).

Apart from market failure arguments, public intervention might also be justified on the grounds that long-term care is regarded as a *merit good* (Musgrave 1959). Even if market failure as described before does not occur with specific goods, they still might be regarded as '... so meritorious that their satisfaction is provided through the public budget, over and above what is provided for through the market and paid for by private buyers.' (Musgrave 1959: 13) However, the concept of merit goods used for justifying state intervention is rather controversial as is the concept itself (Sievering 1996; Berthold 1988).

Whereas market failure and merit goods are concerned with allocation, state intervention may also be justified for distributional reasons. In a for-profit market system resources are allocated according to the consumers' ability and willingness to pay. The outcome of this allocation process may, however, not correspond with distributional or equity objectives in a specific society. But this – which in fact also is true for the existence of market failure – still does not necessarily require state intervention as other institutional settings such as the non-profit sector and the informal sector might fulfil this role.

From an equity perspective these alternative institutional approaches do produce other potential inequities. In the informal sector non-members of the small social community tend to be excluded or at least are not provided with the same amount of resources. The form, the role and the behaviour of non-profit organisations is the result of a complex mixture of features (e.g. Badelt 1998). Equity concerns tend to be at the root of their activities. However, because of the voluntary approach, specific orientations or the lack of funds, this also might result in a distribution of resources which is regarded as inequitable by actors outside these organisations.

Hence, with regard to equity there are potential 'failures' or 'inadequacies' in the various institutional settings which might require state intervention. Relevant issues of state intervention for equity reasons in long-term care are intragenerational and intergenerational distribution, horizontal and vertical distribution, the division between public and private responsibilities as well as territorial distribution. As the issue of equity is at the core of this study, it will be discussed in much more detail in the following sections.

Translating welfare state concerns in welfare state practice is not just a question of efficiency and equity considerations, but a result of the complexity of public choice issues including the role of the electorate, pressure groups, parties, as well as bureaucrats and the valuation of different societal and welfare state objectives by the various actors in the policy making process. Although debates regarding the role of the welfare state are very much about state vs. market, long-term care is a prime example for the much broader institutional mix in welfare, where the role of the public sector varies considerably from general regulation, to financing long-term care services without being the actual provider of services, to the public sector as a service provider.

2.5 Conclusions

Long-term care is about providing and financing care over an extended period of time. The informal, the for-profit, the voluntary (non-profit), and the public sector all may act as, on the one hand, providers of services and – at least as mediators – of financial means and, on the other hand, as financiers of long-term care. Although coverage of long-term care needs requires a considerable amount of resources, long-term care has long been a hidden agenda in most welfare states. Issues that make long-term care increasingly important in the social policy debate, and will do so for at least a couple of decades to come, are demographic changes, socio-economic patterns, incentives from the wider economic and social system, as well as economic constraints in extending publicly financed welfare state benefits.

Recent policy directions in long-term care can be summarised as policies '... to contain the heavy growth of health expenditure, to define policy priorities for the rapidly growing group of elderly persons, to provide adequate coverage for the growing need of long-term care, to reorganise residential care, and to introduce new incentives for the development of community care and informal care.' (Walker, Guillemard, Alber 1993: 62) We might find similar policy measures in many countries incorporating many or some of these policy trends. But, the extent to which they are introduced, whether they emphasise payments or services, how they recognise the role of informal care givers and the way in which they are integrated in the whole welfare system results in considerable differences between countries and even within countries.

As far as equity is concerned, policy statements in long-term care are rather vague – if the term 'equity' is used at all. However, objectives such as 'provision of an adequate coverage' or 'redistribution between public and private responsibility' point at equity considerations in long-term care. The concept, the various interpretations of equity, and the way in which equity is translated into long-term care practice will be analysed in the following parts of this study.

3 Equity and Long-Term Care: A Framework for Analysis

The objective of this part of the study is to conceptualise an analytical tool for the comparative analysis of equity choices in long-term care policies. The focus is on equity as it is translated into practice, that is the various dimensions and interpretations to be found in the realisation of equity through social policies, on how public policies interfere in long-term care systems by providing, financing, and regulating long-term care. The objective of this study is not to analyse the normative question of how equity should be defined in long-term care or to analyse single specific interpretations of equity in long-term care, but to develop a framework covering the range of interpretations of equity to be found in actual long-term care policies.

In the first chapter 3.1 the concept of equity will be introduced showing the variations in using this and related terms such as justice, fairness, and equality. The following chapter 3.2 addresses the question of how equity is analysed in long-term care. This includes a brief review of the literature which will also consider some work in health care, a closely related social policy field. The brief survey shows a considerable lack of research regarding equity concerns as they are translated into practice, which is the main focus of this study.

The basic structure of the approach will be introduced in chapter 3.3 by discussing the main features of equity choices and placing the study in equity research. In chapters 3.4 and 3.5, the approach will be specified and discussed in more detail for the provision of long-term care and the finance of long-term care. The guiding dimensions are three main features: the goods (resources or burdens) to be allocated, among whom to allocate the respective goods (the subjects of allocation), and according to which principles.

3.1 The basic terminology of equity

Equity is widely accepted as an objective in social policy. Explicitly or implicitly, welfare state definitions as well as definitions of social policy include notions such as equity, justice or equality. And equity is an attractive label in social policy making. Equity obviously is one of the key characteristics of any policy approach that attempts to find broad support. However, apart from a basic agreement on equity as an objective of the welfare state, we are far from reaching an agreement on what constitutes equity. Precise specifications of equity are rare in policy-making as well as in research. Hence, equity is sometimes introduced as the elusive issue, as a 'very messy business' (Elster 1992: 15) or as a subject that might not even exist (Young 1994: xi).

In research, very different traditions have developed with regard to equity or justice in various disciplines. As caricatured by Bell, Schoekkart (1992): '... for philosophers it is a problem of moral rightness. For economists, it is a problem of the efficient realization of social choice. For lawyers, it is a problem of conformity to rules. For social psychologists, it is a matter of individual reactions in interpersonal relations. And for sociologists, it is a mixture of all the preceeding points of view. The positions are not necessarily contradictory, but they are not always easy to correlate.'

There is no consensus regarding the differentiation between terms such as equity, justice, or fairness. The same terminology is used for quite different features as well as different terminology often is used synonymously. According to Bell, Schokkaert (1992: 237) justice and equity are a measure of the acceptability of certain features of human relationships or situations. These features include the macro-level of social institutions as well as the micro-level of human relationships, they address procedural issues as well as results, and they include ethical and descriptive approaches. And, justice and equity do address a moral duty, whereas an individual is free to be charitable.

Fairness is often used as a synonym with equity or justice, but even more as a term to describe these features. With regard to the differences between equity and justice, there is a clear distinction made in some disciplines, e.g. in law (Bell 1992). In other disciplines such as in economics, there is no agreement in the use of the two terms, probably most agreement on using them as synonyms (Le Grand 1991).

Here – following the dominance in the actual use of the terms – justice will be used with relation to normative theories of justice. With regard to the objective of this study, they will be touched upon only briefly in chapter 3.2. For an overview of various approaches see e.g. Kolm (1997), Roemer (1998; 1996) and in relation to health Le Grand (1991), Gillon (1986) or Daniels (1985).

Equity – following Young (1994) – will be used for dealing with concrete situations. With regard to long-term care issues, this touches upon a variety of very different questions such as: How does the state intervene in the design of long-term care systems? To what extent are services allocated according to need? Which definition of need is used for the allocation of services? According to what principles are payments for care distributed? How does the state allocate the burdens of financing long-term care? What approaches can be used to analyse the effectiveness of these equity interpretations?

A further important distinction has to be made between equity and equality. Whereas equity covers the full range of acceptable real features of human relationships and situations, equality deals with specific interpretations (Le Grand 1991). For example, equity in long-term care may be defined as 'equal use of long-term care services according to need' or as 'equal use of long-term care services according to contributions paid'. These are only two different interpretations of equity, both situations might be seen as equitable, but would certainly result in considerable differences in the actual distribution of long-term care services. Following the first principle ('equality according to need') implies inequality according to contributions paid, and vice versa. Equitable outcomes may be seen as unequal and vice versa.

3.2 Studying equity in long-term care – A survey of the literature

Searching for equity studies in long-term care is an almost fruitless task. There are important exceptions, but most studies – and this is true for other areas in social policy as well – address very specific interpretations of equity, other studies are locally restricted, or include only one type of service provision within the complex arena of the existing modes of delivery. Generally, specifications of what is meant by equity or an equitable allocation in long-term care are rare. Existing specifications often seem to be based on a mixture of what is supposed to be a widely accepted interpretation and what is going to be testable, given the data available. As research on equity issues in long-term care is rather limited, the following brief survey will also consider studies from other social policy fields, in particular from health care, sharing a number of characteristics with long-term care.

First of all, the issue of equity is at the core of the debate on theories of justice. For an overview see among others Kolm (1997), Roemer (1996), Scherer (1992), Barry (1989) or – with regard to their role in health care –

Gillon (1986). With regard to their design theories of justice can be differentiated according to three dimensions (Dobson 1998): 'Impartiality' vs. 'substantiveness' is '... whether any given theory of justice should be impartial in respect to notions of the good for human beings, or whether it should be read off from, or even be in the service of, the given notion of the good.' (Dobson 1998: 69) The second dimension is about whether a situation is just, because the procedure to achieve that situation was just ('procedural justice') or whether the outcome per se is regarded as just ('consequentialist justice'). Finally, theories of justice are either designed as a theory of universally applicable principles or as a theory that argues for principles that are related to specific historical, societal and cultural modes (Walzer 1983).

With regard to the principles underlying the various theories of justice, the libertarian and the collectivist egalitarian approach can be seen as two opposite approaches. In the libertarian view, access to and the use of health and long-term care follows the market principle. Health care is allocated and distributed according to demand and supply of such services, it becomes part of the reward system of that society. Variations according to income and wealth are part of the libertarian 'outcome'. By contrast, in the egalitarian view, need should be the only criterion according to which access to and use of health care are determined.

Another approach to categorise theories of justice focuses on the 'object' of equalisation (following Fleurbaey 1995), without denying most important differences between various authors in the respective bundles which, however, can not be discussed here. Some authors, such as Dworkin (1981a, 1981b) or Rawls (1971) are focusing at equalising resources. In Rawls' theory, for example, resources to be equalised are the so-called primary goods. Others, such as Roemer (1986), Arneson (1989), Cohen (1989) or Sen (1985) are emphasising equality of opportunities. Sen, for example, in his theory of justice aims at equalising basic capabilities enabling individuals to translate resources into functionings. Finally, theories of justice might be aimed at outcome, such as the Fleurbaey approach of equalising social outcome (Fleurbaey 1995).

More recently there is increasing interest in theories of justice and health care and the applicability of different approaches to health care (e.g. Le Grand 1991; Gillon 1986; Daniels 1985; Peirera 1993). The range of choices open to individuals is at the heart of the Le Grand approach. 'Situations where one person is disadvantaged relative to another due to factors beyond either's control are commonly judged inequitable; situations where the disadvantage arises because of differences in individual choices freely made are not. Equity depends on the extent of individual choice.' (Le

Grand 1991: 176) Applying this to the health care system, Le Grand argues for health care that is free at the point of use. If health risks for oneself or others are identifiable as an individual's responsibility they should pay a hypothecated tax rather than be made liable for all costs arising at the point of use. Daniel's main argument in his theory of justice in the distribution of health care is that health care has crucial effects on equality of opportunity. '... shares of the normal range will be *fair* when positive steps have been taken to make sure that individuals maintain normal functioning, where possible, and that there are no other discriminatory impediments to their choice of life plans.' (Daniels 1985: 57)

With regard to long-term care, the existence of handicaps and long-term care needs is ignored in many of these normative approaches. For example, following Rawls' principle of an equal distribution of primary goods would provide handicapped people with exactly the same amount of these goods than non-handicapped people, as was shown in the critique by Sen (1982) or Rothstein (1998). Jacobs (1993) in her critique points out that handicaps – in Dworkin's approach – are reduced to the effect they have on income in a market economy.

Daniels (1985) in his work on theories of justice and health care addresses the question of whether ageing and care for the elderly pose a distinct distribution problem. While discussing equal opportunity with regard to different requirements in different stages of life, Daniels argues for age-relative opportunity ranges. '... justice requires we allocate health care in a manner that assures individuals a fair chance at enjoying the normal opportunity range, and prudence suggests that it is equally important to protect individual opportunity range for each stage of life.' (Daniels 1985: 112)

A second research strand is focusing on 'what the people think' (Miller 1992). Whereas theories of justice presented before are searching for an ideal interpretation of justice, these empirical studies are searching for beliefs and judgements regarding social justice as well as causes and consequences of such judgements. (For an overview to this approach see among others Törnblom 1992 or Miller 1992.) Judgements may refer to institutions, procedures or outcomes, they may refer to distributions in personal relationships and smaller communities as well as to societal distributions (e.g. Montada, Lerner 1996; Lerner, Mikula 1994). For long-term care, intra-family distributions are of considerable importance. Despite extended public intervention, long-term care is still very much a family or household responsibility. Among other factors, active or reactive decisions regarding the allocation of resources and burdens are influenced by social justice judgements (Reichle 1996; Mikula 1998). Overall, studies clearly show that principles of social justice codetermine the allocation and division of resources and burdens. There are, however, considerable variations in the perception of justice and, hence, in the response to this valuation with factors such as cultural and socio-economic background, values and attitudes, gender, class, the resources or burdens to be allocated, the subjects involved, etc. (Törnblom 1992).

The third stream of literature deals with the analysis of outcomes. It is studied to what extent empirical distributions correspond with specific interpretations of equity. In health care there is a wide range of studies addressing questions of this type. Department of Health (1998), Fox (1989) or van Doorslaer, Wagstaff, Bleichrodt, et al. (1997) are examining equality in the distribution of health. Despite all the efforts and the success of public health care systems, these studies show considerable inequalities in health among different socio-economic groups. A strong association was found between inequalities in income and inequalities in health which is particularly high in the United Kingdom, and lowest in Sweden, Finland and the former East Germany (van Doorslaer, Wagstaff, Bleichrodt, et al. 1997).

Le Grand (1982) studies the distribution of public expenditure and the respective impact for various policy areas including health and social services. The analysis is based on five different interpretations of equity: equality of public expenditure, equality of final income, equality of use, equality of cost (costs of using the service) and equality of outcome. Le Grand concludes that public expenditure has not achieved equality in any of these dimensions, in some respects not even reduced inequalities. Instead, inequalities have been rather persistent over time.

The study by van Doorslaer, Wagstaff, Rutten (1993) – as well as a series of subsequent studies (e.g. van Doorslaer, Wagstaff, van der Burg, et al. 1999) – does not just look at the provision of health care, but also includes the finance of health care offering a broad picture of the distributional implications of the design of health care systems in a comparative perspective. In the provision of care, inequalities in morbidity and variations of health expenditure across income groups according to age, sex and morbidity are tested. Analysing equity in the finance of health care in this study is based on measuring progressivity of the respective financing system. The study uses specific interpretations of equity in health care receiving broad public support. But the quantitative analysis does not take into account to what extent these equity concerns differ across countries. The study shows that in the finance of care the actual degree and direction of redistributional effects depends on the mix in the revenue system, with direct taxes being at least slightly progressive, indirect taxes and social insurance contributions being regressive and private payments being highly regressive. For the delivery of health care, overall, there is no clear evidence that care received depends on income. Even so, this is the fact for aspects of the system such as specialist treatment in some countries.

Overall, most empirical equity studies in social policy spend considerably more effort on analysing certain specific interpretations of equity than on analysing to what extent these interpretations are relevant with regard to explicit or implicit health policy objectives, to what extent other interpretations of equity might give a quite different picture of equity in health care, or to what extent they correspond with theories of social justice.

Again, in long-term care the number of studies of this type is rather small. Exceptions are the studies by Davies, Fernández, Nomer (2000), Davies, Fernández, Saunders (1998), Evandrou, Falkingham, Le Grand, Winter (1992) and Bebbington, Davies (1983). Bebbington and Davies are investigating equity in the receipt of home help with regard to sex discrimination and territorial distribution of home help services. The concept they are using is that of target efficiency, that is the '... efficiency with which a service is targeted on and among those persons judged to be the most appropriate benefactors.' (Bebbington, Davies 1983: 310f) Evandrou, et al. analyse the distribution of primary health care and domiciliary care for elderly people. In their study a distribution is defined as equitable if '... only variables which measure respondent's need for the service provide a significant explanation of whether the respondent receives the service.' (Evandrou, Falkingham, Le Grand, Winter 1992: 489) Both studies point out that need is a significant determinant in the use of social services but not the only determinant. According to the evidence of the two studies, the actual distribution does not correspond with what was defined as an equitable distribution.

Davies, Fernández, Nomer (2000) and Davies, Fernández, Saunders (1998) represent only most recent publications from a bundle of related publications on community care for elderly people by Davies and others. The publications build on the production of welfare approach (see Knapp 1984; Davies, Knapp 1981) and a broad collection of evidence in the UK, and more recently in France. In Davies, Fernández, Nomer (2000) the implications of variations in service inputs on outcomes with regard to users and care givers are studied. Apart from an in-depth investigation of efficiencies with regard to a range of indicator variables such as length of stay in the community, user satisfaction and dissatisfaction, etc., the study also searches for implicit equity judgements with regard to output variables. Length of stay in the community is the most significantly valued output, whereas other priorities differ considerably depending on underlying assumptions in the scenarios used in the study. Need-related circumstances and actual service allocation is at the core of the study by Davies, Fernández, Saunders (1998). It is investigated how need-related circumstances correspond with service allocation and how this changes over time. The study offers detailed evidence from various sites in France and the United Kingdom showing quite considerable differences in need-related circumstances and the actual use of home and community services between the two countries. The major focus of research by Davies and others is on the production of welfare approach and actual decisions resulting from interactions and negotiations between care managers, users and care givers. With regard to equity concerns, the interest in allocating resources in long-term care and the respective consequences for equity are on the micro-level, whereas the research presented in this book focuses on the meso-level of welfare state design (see figure 3.1).

Summing up, there is increasing interest in theories of justice and health care and there is increasing evidence of the distribution of specific goods or resources regarding specific interpretations of equity. On the other hand, there is a lack of research dealing with the question of the 'empirical rules of equity', of equity choices, the interpretations of equity to be found in practice. '... there have been virtually no attempts to study the whole range of questions of this kind, and to develop a conceptual and theoretical framework to describe and explain how institutions allocate goods and burdens.' (Elster 1992)

Prominent exceptions are Young (1994), Elster (1992) and Rae (1981), studying equity considerations as they are found in the real world. The work by Rae (1981) is a study of the 'grammar of equality' conceptualising the way equality concerns are transformed from theory into practice. The study by Young (1994) is on the meaning of equity in concrete everyday situations. He argues that equity is the outcome of competing principles of need, desert and social utility what is then discussed in a variety of case studies. Elster (1992) deals with 'local justice', studying the mechanisms of allocating resources, the implications of specific principles, and how the selection of specific principles might be explained. All three studies do not focus on specific issues, but are full of examples from different spheres of real life, including issues such as kidney transplantations, language rights, progressive taxation, the assignment of students to dormitories, access to higher education, etc. The different spheres are the main focus of the work of Walzer (1983), whose approach however – other than in the studies just mentioned – is normative suggesting a pluralistic theory of justice.

Calabresi, Bobbit (1978), Lee (1996), Schmidt, Hartmann (1997) or Engelstad (1994) are examples for studying equity in the allocation of specific goods. The latter two publications are following the concept of local justice (Elster 1992) by analysing the allocation of specific goods such as layoffs, kidneys in transplant medicine or access to universities. Calabresi and Bobbit (1978) are focusing on tragic choices, for example, in the allocation of dialysis, analysing allocation according to four major principles: allocation via the market, allocation according to political decisions, according to lotteries and according to the 'evolutionary' approach. The study by Lee (1996) is focused on educational issues. He explores what equity looks like in the funding of additional educational needs under the Local Management of Schools. The study, including four case studies, also analyses causal factors for the actual allocation and the implications of respective decisions. All these studies are showing that interpretations of equity, as revealed by choices made in the various policy areas, are much more complex than any single normative approach or any single interpretation of equity.

In this study, the analysis of equity choices in long-term care follows Young (1994) and Elster (1992) in their interest in how equity concerns look in the real world, literature on the design of welfare policies (e.g. Gilbert, Specht, Terrell 1993), and the public economics literature (see e.g. Stiglitz 2000; Cullis, Jones 1998) regarding the design of expenditure and taxation programmes. The sphere it focuses on is long-term care. In contrast to Lee (1996) – focusing on a specific resource in education – or Calabresi and Bobbit (1978) – focusing on a specific type of goods, namely tragic choices – this study is focusing on a social policy area, long-term care needs and the public response to the occurrence of such needs. Long-term care needs might be covered by various resources and financed from different sources with welfare state intervention and its potential choices being one possible response. Before proceeding with a more detailed elaboration of a framework for analysis, some general remarks on features of equity choices in long-term care have to be made.

3.3 The concept of 'equity choices'

Some main features of equity choices

Choices in the allocation of resources and burdens take place at different societal levels and within different institutional settings (Young 1994; Elster 1992). Choices have to be made or might be made in the public sector and in the formal private sector as well as in the informal sector (see chapter 2.3; Evers, Olk 1996; Gough 1993). Choices and decisions to be made in terms of equity do, however, differ quite considerably in the various sectors. In the private for-profit sector, allocation and distribution are guided by the price mechanism. This system provides the basis to produce and to allocate goods according to preferences, ability and willingness-to-pay. Under the ideal assumptions, the resulting resource allocation will be efficient and – according to a specific interpretation of equity – equitable. But equity concerns themselves are no guiding principle in the allocation.

Allocation by the state sector – in a democratic system – is based on individuals voting for representatives. These representatives, in turn, vote for a public budget and decide whether or not, how and to what extent the public sector takes responsibility for long-term care. The allocation itself, including the fine-steering of principles, is undertaken by hierarchically structured administrative agencies. Here, equity concerns do play a major role even if the definition of equity objectives often tends to be rather vague (see chapter 4.2).

The non-profit sector is a rather heterogeneous sector which makes the identification of an ideal model a rather difficult task. Efforts to describe access to the goods provided by the non-profit sector and the principles used to allocate goods emphasise the concepts of needs and solidarity. What makes the non-profit sector distinct from the public sector is that covering specific needs is not and can not be guaranteed as a legal or as a social right, even so non-profit organisations might represent a very important lobby for specifying such rights in society.

The informal sector, finally, is defined as a small social community, such as families, households or the neighbourhood. Apart from being part of this social community the allocation of goods is determined by a mixture of principles including such notions as altruism, reciprocity, trust, etc.

As mentioned before, these are just four basic social institutions involved in the production of welfare. More recently, developments are characterised by an increasing mix of welfare sectors. For example, by splitting the role of purchaser (state sector) and provider (private sector) in the delivery of social services or by state intervention in the informal sector offering social insurance coverage to informal care givers without establishing regular employment relationships.

Within all these institutional settings, choices have to be made on different levels. Calabresi, Bobbit (1978) distinguish first-order and second-order decisions by pointing at the determination of the overall amount of a specific good to be produced and at the determination of who shall get what share of it. Here, following Young (1994), three levels shall be distinguished: macro-level, meso-level and micro-level choices or decisions. On the macro-level, choices have to be made regarding the total amount of resources or burdens to be allocated. For the public sector, how much of the public budget to spend on long-term care issues is the question. Long-term care, hence, competes with all other public responsibilities in social policy and beyond.

These macro choices, however, also occur in the private formal as well as informal sphere. Organisations in the formal private sector subsidised by public bodies through global budgets may have to make such decisions. In the informal private sphere the decision is on how to use family or household budgets for competing wants.

Though macro-level choices are not the major focus of this study, the issues of intergenerational equity and age-biases in social policy should be briefly addressed here. Given financial restrictions and socio-demographic trends (see chapter 2.2), the debate on the design of welfare state policies is increasingly focused on the generational division of welfare and more general on the allocation of resources among competing policy fields. With regard to long-term care needs, this is, on the one hand, about the relative importance of long-term care compared to prevention, acute care and rehabilitation and about whether there are age-related considerations. These questions are to be found in the debates about how to define and how to promote health and well-being as well as issues concerning rationing in health and social care (Moody 1998; Binstock, Post 1991; Smeeding 1987). On the other hand, macro choices have to be made with regard to benefits for different age-groups. Whether or not, how and to what extent the public sector intervenes in caring obligations regarding children, the disabled and the frail elderly constitutes a specific distribution of the respective burdens. Evaluating equity in this respect requires not just age as a criterion – which in itself is quite controversial – but a consideration of a variety of variables including the historical, social and cultural context as well as the long-term effects of the distribution at a certain point in time (see e.g. Sgritta 1994; Daniels 1988).

The second type of choices and decisions, which will be called meso-level choices, take place when the total amount of resources or burdens has to be allocated among 'eligible' individuals or parties. From a welfare state perspective decisions to be made include, for example, the decision whether to provide cash benefits or in-kind benefits, the establishment of entitlement criteria, etc. The meso-level is the main focus of the study and will be discussed in detail below and in the following chapters 3.4 and 3.5

regarding the provision (allocating resources) and the finance (allocating burdens) of long-term care.

Finally, on the micro-level individuals react to these decisions by adapting their behaviour and their own allocation principles. For example, individuals might change their attitudes towards informal care-giving as a response to the changing role of the state in long-term care provision. Consequently, what amount and what kind of care finally is received by the individual in need of care is not just the result of a single allocation decision, but the result of a number of such decisions on different societal levels.

Allocation decisions in real life are not made once and for all. Rae (1981), using the term 'equalities', and Lee (1996), using the term 'equities', are pointing at the dynamic concept of equality and equity. Situations regarded as equal or unequal or as equitable or inequitable at one point in time are constantly challenged by the social, economic and political environment. The famous 'equality – efficiency tradeoff' (Okun 1975) is a prominent example for this dynamic process.

Existing equity rules may also be challenged by the quality of specific resources which determines the allocation of resources in a number of ways. Principles of allocation for homogenous and divisible resources are not necessarily appropriate for the allocation of inhomogeneous or indivisible goods. Money – a resource that can be used in the finance of care and as an intermediate good in the provision of care – can be divided into almost indefinitely small shares without reducing the quality of these shares. With indivisible resources – such as places in nursing homes – partition would destroy the quality of the resource.

Another important issue related to the quality of the resources is the differentiation between what is actually allocated and what this allocation is aimed at. Elster (1992: 186) identifies three types of goods according to the possibility to equalise their distribution: 'First, there are goods which can be allocated, like money, material goods, and services. Second, there are goods that cannot be allocated, but whose distribution can be affected by the allocations of other goods. The distribution of self-respect, welfare, knowledge, or health depends largely on the allocation of money, goods, and services. Third, there are mental and physical capacities whose distribution cannot be affected by allocation, because they are determined genetically or are subject to irreversible accidents (such as the loss of a limb).'

In long-term care all three types of goods are relevant, those that can be allocated (type I goods), those whose distribution can be affected through allocating other goods (type II goods) and those whose distribution cannot be affected through allocation (type III goods). This characteristic of long-term care related goods, among other features (see chapter 2.3), is one of the reasons for the complexity and the specific feature of long-term care. Disabled people who are unable to participate in the labour market are faced with a lack of income opportunity, a type I goods problem. Re-allocation in this case can be undertaken by just re-allocating the goods in question, that is money.

But the example just mentioned is not only about replacing income. Apart from being unable to acquire certain goods, disabled as well as frail elderly people often will suffer from losing self-respect, from being restricted in their ability to live independently. Self-respect and independent living are examples of the type II goods. They cannot be re-allocated directly. However, it is possible to re-allocate other goods. Supported employment programmes, social services, or payments to buy assistance are only three possibilities of how the distribution of type II goods might be affected in the desired direction.

The specific characteristic of type II goods has received some considerable attention in the economics literature on the production of health and social care (e.g. Knapp 1984). The final outcome in social care are concepts like health (which is restricted in long-term care compared to the traditional health care system), well-being or quality of life. Because of practicality problems, the focus on actual equity rules tends to be on intermediate rather than final outputs, that is care. The implications of shifting from final to intermediate outputs can be shown by a small example: Two people, A and B, with exactly the same physical restrictions, provided with exactly the same intermediate output, might experience quite different final outputs. Take the example of A and B, both restricted in their ability to walk independently outside their own house. For A walking is a necessary movement to do shopping. For B it is more than that; B enjoys walking. If both A and B are supported by social services in shopping, B compared to A is going to have a smaller increase in well-being by the same service.

Finally, there are type III goods, one of the key characteristics of long-term care. People in need of long-term care suffer from an irreversible lack of certain abilities or functionings. This cannot be equalised. The only approach is to compensate for this, with at least two possibilities of such compensation. To some extent the lack of certain abilities can be replaced by an alternative functioning, for example through wheelchairs. But this can never be a full replacement and sometimes there is no such alternative available. Here, compensation can only be offered in the form of goods that are not connected to the ability or the functioning the person lacks. An example of such compensation is a disability benefit.

The distribution of a specific good may support the distribution of goods type I, II and III at the same time. A disability benefit, for example, might be seen as income replacement, it might be seen as a means to buy services in the care market, as a means to improve individual well-being or as a compensation for the disability. Using the three types is a helpful construct for discussing objectives and means of long-term care policies, but it does not provide a basic structure to analyse equity choices.

Placing the framework in equity research

The focus of this study is on the analysis of equity choices in the design of long-term care policies in a comparative perspective. Equity is not treated as an abstract conception, but as choices as they appear in actual efforts to allocate resources and burdens.

An abstract description of the issues embedded in this approach can be found in the following definition of equity: 'a certain amount of x to each y according to z', reflecting the three main characteristics according to which interpretations of equity may differ. The three features are: WHAT is to be shared (x – the goods to be shared, the object of allocation), between WHOM (y – the subject of allocation), and HOW (z – according to which principle). Again, the agreement on this basic definition is widespread. However, questions such as what resources to allocate, how to assess what are equitable shares of the respective resources or burdens, to what extent to differentiate among unequals, how to define the allocation principle, etc. make the analysis of equity choices most controversial. In many equity studies there is not much effort on explicitly discussing these questions. Exceptions regarding conceptual discussion and empirical investigation of at least some of these characteristics can be found in Lee (1996); Gilbert, Specht, Terrell (1993); Sen (1992); Elster (1992); Le Grand (1991, 1982). The following analysis explores the three characteristics of equity choices for long-term care policies following the distinction between the provision and the finance of long-term care. In the provision of care the focus will be on how the welfare state intervenes in the allocation of care resources. In analysing equity choices in the finance of long-term care the study looks at the role of the welfare state in designing respective equity choices. Particular attention will be paid to the way informal care givers are addressed in long-term care policies, which are all too often completely ignored in the analysis of allocational and distributional issues in the finance of the welfare state.

The study concentrates on the meso-level of welfare state choices, that is the actual decisions that have to be made to design the allocation of resources and burdens in long term care (see Table 3.1). Decisions regarding the overall amount of resources made available (macro-level) as well as the reactions to the respective decisions on the micro-level are not the main focus, but will be touched upon in the discussion, in particular with regard to implicit allocation principles.

Table 3.1 Equity choices on the macro-, meso- and micro-level

Macro-level	*Meso-level*	*Micro-level*
Choices and decisions regarding the overall amount of resources	Choices and decisions regarding what (the specific resource to be shared), among whom (the focal units) and how (according to which principles)	Choices and decisions regarding the actual behaviour, including the reaction to choices made on the macro-level, the meso-level and on the micro-level

Before proceeding with these issues a further clarification of terminology is necessary. Terminology might be clear-cut if approaching an issue just from one disciplinary focus, but not – as it is the case with this study – if research is characterised by an interdisciplinary approach. The concept of equity is a good example for this predicament. Here, the term 'equity choices' is used to point at the choices that are available and the decisions that have to be made, when resources, rights, burdens, costs, etc. are allocated. In this context 'equity rules' or 'interpretations of equity' will be used to indicate potential or actual choices made. Allocation is the assignment of these goods to specific individuals, groups, institutions or other communities. The study follows a basic distinction between the provision and the finance of care. The goods to be allocated in the provision of long-term care will be called resources, covering in-kind services, cash benefits as well as rights or rules in the provision of care set by the state as the regulatory body. Burdens are the goods or costs to be allocated in the finance of long-term care, including again cash and in-kind contributions as well as duties.

3.4 Equity and the allocation of resources

Long-term care is about providing help, assistance and support to those people in need of care. As has been shown in the second part of this study, the provision of care can be organised in various institutional settings in the informal as well as in the formal sector and can take different forms of delivery.

The interest here is how the state intervenes in choices regarding the provision of care, be it in the role as a supplier of care (either as purchaser or as actual provider) or in the role as a regulatory body. The analysis is focused on equity choices with regard to the implications on those in need of care, that is potential care receivers. However, state intervention in the provision of care does not only affect care receivers. State intervention creates incentives in the entire care environment, including formal and informal structures. For example, the welfare mix and the role of non-profit organisations will look quite different depending on whether non-profit organisations act as providers who are financed mainly by state subsidies or in an environment where their finance is based on fees, donations and voluntary work. Similarly, incentives might be created for the informal and the formal for-profit sector, making arrangements in these welfare sectors more or less 'attractive'. Equities or inequities among these intermediate actors are not the major focus of the analysis, but will however be looked at as far as they are the intermediate focus of welfare state intervention.

The resources to be shared

The first issue according to which interpretations of equity may differ is the resource to be shared. This seems to be a rather clear issue. But, an equitable allocation in long-term care is not only about allocating care, it is about support in activities of daily living, compensating for inabilities, self-respect, independent living, etc. Obviously, a more systematic examination of the good or the goods to be shared in the provision of long-term care is necessary.

Social policy is aimed at improving social and/or economic conditions or life chances of individuals or groups within society. Consequently, it seems appropriate to look at the *final outcome* of long-term care provision. Outcome in long-term care – broadly understood – is the impact or the effect of long-term care-giving on those in need of care and potential effects on others involved in the process of care-giving, such as informal carers. Specific measures of the final outcome, such as the ability to stay in one's own home, are relatively easy to assess. An assessment of overall measures of the final outcome, such as *well-being*, health or welfare, is confronted with enormous conceptual and practical problems (Nocon, Qureshi 1998; Gibson 1998), apart from the ethical question of whether and to what extent it is a public responsibility to equalise welfare levels across individuals (Putterman, Roemer, Silvestre 1998).

The measurement of outcome might include notions of subjective as well as objective quality. Whereas objective quality measures, such as single vs. double or triple bedrooms in nursing homes, tend to be close to concepts measuring service quality and not the actual satisfaction with the outcome of the service, subjective measures – such as empowerment or autonomy – are confronted with severe problems of measurement and generalisation. A further distinction can be made between the assessment by professionals and by users. Evidence shows that views vary quite considerably between professionals and users, among different groups of professionals as well as between users and informal carers (see Nocon, Qureshi 1996).

The final outcome in long-term care is an example for goods whose distribution can not be arranged directly through allocation policies. (see chapter 3.3) Long-term care policies therefore might be more concerned with the 'intermediate output' (Davies, Knapp 1981; Knapp 1984). Here, the focus is on *use* of long-term care in quantitative and qualitative terms. Use or treatment has been the focus of a number of studies on equity in social policy (e.g. Evandrou, Falkingham, Le Grand, Winter 1992; van Doorslaer, Wagstaff, Rutten 1993), partly because this is what policies are aimed at explicitly, partly for reasons of practicality in the assessment of actual use. (Re)allocation of intermediate outputs does not necessarily mean equalisation in the outcome (see the example in chapter 3.3), but may still be seen as equitable.

If the egalitarian objective of equalising resources is reduced in favour of a more liberal approach concerned with the choice of individuals, a third approach has to be introduced, *access*. Access does not necessarily expand choice among potential users, it does however – compared to allocating use – put more weight on the concept of individual freedom leaving more room for self-determined preferences. Access is the opportunity to use specific long-term care services, including the opportunity not to use them. It may be interpreted as the opportunity to get access to a special service, the opportunity to get information on services available, the opportunity to get access to help within a certain amount of time, etc. Policies aimed at equalising access are aimed at equalising potential, not actual use of services. Here, society is not interested whether or not and to what extent frail elderly or disabled people are really cared for or supported.

The potential interpretations of access already point at measurement problems involved. One approach to measure access is by assessing the costs of getting access: '... equal access means that two (or more) individuals face the same costs to themselves of using the health care facility ...' (Mooney 1992: 104) Cost usually does not cover the range of choice, which also could be seen as part of the concept of access.

Widening the concept of access to specific services to a concept of access to a range of potential services addresses *choice*. For example, a system offering places in nursing homes to everyone might fulfil the concept of access to nursing homes, choice, however, remains rather restricted if social services are limited. Individuals might be restricted in choice, either because of a lack of resources or because of factors or preferences beyond their control. Public policies aimed at widening choice, therefore, might take two rather distinct forms. Public policies providing additional monetary resources enable recipients to freely choose how to use these resources. If, in that case, the public sector does not take any additional regulatory measures, the actual allocation and distribution will follow reactive decisions on the individual level including a broad range of variables such as the informational background, individual preferences or values. If, however, there is a societal interest in the kind and the quality of care that is allocated, choice sets will take a different form. Either by regulating the use of financial resources provided (e.g. restricting it to buying services on the formal market), by providing vouchers (Nocera, Zweifel 1996; Eger, Weise 1998) or by providing in-kind services instead of cash benefits. In this case, choice still remains high on the policy agenda, but is combined with an interest in the actual allocation of care.

What actually is allocated is not final outcome, use, access or choice per se, but use of, access to or choice among specific resources. These resources are in-kind services including social services, places as well as services in residential care settings, and care in the informal sector. Other resources that might be allocated are vouchers or money. These intermediate resources then can be used to receive in-kind services just mentioned. Finally, the state has the opportunity to 'design' use of, access to and choice of provision by regulating institutional settings other than the public sector. This might include, for example, the obligation for non-profit organisations to offer care to individuals characterised by specific needs if these non-profit organisations are subsidised by the state. Another example for the regulatory role would be an obligation for family care to be found in social assistance schemes in a number of European countries.

The subjects of resource allocation

The second characteristic feature to investigate different interpretations of equity are the units among which the resources are to be shared. The subjects in the provision of care are individuals in need of care. But policies may also address broader units, such as families or households, geographical areas, nations or institutions.

Equity across *geographical areas* signifies the equitable allocation of goods between local areas, regions, nations, or even beyond. For example, quality standards, such as a certain number of home nurses related to the total population, set by the central government for the development of social services on the local level are aimed at territorial justice as is the allocation of national funds for the development of services on the local level according to the availability of services in this area. *Institutions* are another focal unit, which – with the introduction of contracting-out models – tend to become even more important. Here, quality standards may also be used to equalise quality levels across providers. In order to promote service provision by a certain institutional mix, resources may be transferred to different institutional forms. Finally, *families* or other informal networks might be approached, for example, with regard to legal obligations to care between family members.

Focal units apart from the individual in need of care are approached as an intermediate focal unit in order to improve the situation of individuals within these areas and supported by these institutions. But focal units other than those in need of care are approached not just as intermediate focal units but also as final focal units. Examples from the long-term care field include labour market regulations or the role of volunteers in non-profit organisations.

In the next section the principles according to which resources can be shared will be analysed. It has to be noted that socio-economic groups – a categorisation particularly important for policy analysis – have not been introduced as a focal unit here. This is because the categorisation of individuals according to certain characteristics already represents a principle according to which resources may be shared.

The principles of allocating resources

Finally, interpretations of equity are characterised by the principle according to which the allocation takes place. There are a number of approaches to categorise such principles, those who offer mutually exclusive categories (as Walzer 1983) or those who search for an exhaustive list of such principles (as Elster 1992). In light of the practical problems of the first approach and the objective to clarify and to systematise the range of interpretations, the following discussion presents various sets of principles that can be used in the allocation of scarce long-term care resources. Apart from need, which is probably the most attractive principle for health and social care issues, these sets of principles include egalitarian, time-related, status, economic, and other principles.

Need seems to be the most adequate allocation principle with respect to equity considerations in the provision of health and social care. If equity is defined as 'equal access for equal need', need is the respect to which individuals are unequal and to which differentiation among individuals should be made. Other variables such as age, gender, or income should not make any difference in access.

However, the concept of need in itself is probably as complex and as 'elusive' as that of equity. A brief overview was given in chapter 2.3 pointing to different interpretations of need, ideas behind the concepts of need and demand as well as approaches to develop a theory of human needs (Doyal, Gough 1991).

For the purposes of this study, need will be used as the term related to limitations or inabilities arising from health problems, and its subsequent requirements regarding care and support. Need as used in the context of this study does not include need due to financial restrictions or because of the lack of close family members who might act as care givers. These aspects will be treated as additional potential criteria of allocation.

But even in the more specific health related context, need is far from being a clear-cut single principle. In benefit schemes as well as in policy analysis or in theoretical considerations of need, one can find a variety of very different measures of need, such as morbidity or disability measures, measures based on the ability to benefit, the inability to carry out certain activities of daily living, or the amount of time required to help people. In addition, it makes a difference whether we rely on self-reported needs or on the assessment by professionals. In any case, the concept of need implies a judgement or an idea about what defines need and what does not. Although the definition of need is central to designing and analysing social policies, there is a significant lack of information on how different interpretations and different assessment procedures do influence the actual outcome of policies (Percy-Smith 1996).

Need has been introduced with a focus on the individual. But society might not only be interested in the needs of individuals. Society may as well be interested in the needs of certain socio-economic groups. In this case the principle of need has to be accompanied by other principles, for example age or occupational status. Obviously, principles used for allocating resources are not necessarily used as single principles, but – and this in fact is almost the rule – as mixed principles.

The idea of *egalitarian principles* is that resources have to be shared equally. Here 'egalitarian' shall be used to name a distribution that does not involve any segmentation among citizens. Every citizen has to get the same amount of the resource to be shared. This might be used as an ideal objective (or as a reference point) for the 'final output' of well-being. Allocating equal shares of care (taking use as the resource to be shared) without considering different levels of disability, however, does not seem an appropriate principle. Above all, because it does not reflect individual needs and because goods involved in the caring process are not infinitely divisible goods.

Time-related principles – in particular waiting-lists and queuing (see e.g. Tietzel, Müller 1998 or – for an empirical investigation – Martin, Smith 1999) – are frequently used in health and long-term care because of their advantages regarding practicality. Waiting lists are fairly common to allocate places to nursing homes, queuing is a method to allocate services. Waiting lists as well as queuing may not only be favoured because of practicality reasons, but also as an indicator of the intensity of needs. At the same time they may reflect the level of information, which questions this principle as an indicator of need. Another form of time-related principle is used in insurance models, if benefits are (partly) related to the duration of time over which contributions are paid.

The set of *status principles* includes a variety of principles such as age, gender, civil status, family status, residence status or occupational status. In health and social care some of these principles are used as an additional principle to define the target group. For example, people might be excluded from medical treatment by age, or places in nursing homes may be reserved for those who are residents within a geographical area. Apart from being used as allocation principles, status variables as well as income (see below) are important in policy analysis to evaluate the effects of welfare state programmes on socio-economic groups.

The typical example for the use of *economic variables* in allocating resources in long-term care is means-testing. For example, benefits or free services are provided to those people in need of care whose income is below a certain level. Apart from income economic variables might include a number of other properties, such as savings or other assets as well as income and assets from close family members. In social assistance schemes, for example, people being cared for in nursing homes are obliged to use their pensions and savings before public bodies interfere.

If different forms of providing care result in the same outcome, efficiency could be an appropriate principle to decide which kind of production to support or which kind of goods to actually provide. Although the outcome of caring for frail elderly people in acute hospitals, in residential care settings or in the community will not be exactly the same, there is room for allocating resources among these different institutions according to the efficiency principle. Indeed, this is one of the driving forces for the redesign of long-term care systems in many countries.

Most of the principles described are not used as single principles, but as *mixed principles*. For example, allocation formulae such as 'payments for care according to a specific definition of need for those 60 years and over' or 'free access to services according to specific definitions of need and income.'

Still, even in case of complex allocation principles there tends to be room for discretionary decisions or principles that are not explicitly stated in the allocation formulae. Here, *'implicit principles'* will be used as additional principles alongside explicit principles introduced before. For example, if people in need of care have to make flat-rate out-of-pocket payments to get access to social services, this might exclude the poorest because of lack of purchasing power. The guiding principle in the private market becomes an implicit additional principle in long-term care policies. The informational background of users, values of individual decision-makers, lobbying and political power or informal connections are further examples for implicit principles in the allocation of resources. An indication of the importance of these 'principles' are non-take-up ratios or variations in the take-up ratio according to socio-economic variables (see e.g. van Oorschot 1991).

Table 3.2 Choices in the provision of long-term care

WHAT (resources)	outcome use access choice *by means of* payments services regulation
WHOM (subjects)	individuals families / households institutions geographical areas
HOW (principles)	need egalitarian time-related status economic mixed implicit

Apart from defining the target group, principles also determine the amount of resources allocated. Take the example of 'equal use according to need'. If A and B are equal in their needs, then they should get the same amount of treatment. If A and B are unequal, they should get an unequal amount. To what extent they should be treated unequally in order to reach an equitable distribution is part of the allocation principle.

Table 3.2 summarises the interpretations of equity in the provision of long-term care. The potential resources to be shared in long-term care are final outputs (well-being), the consumption of intermediate outputs (use), access and choice. The social policy means to achieve an equitable distribution in these resources are regulation, in-kind resources or cash payments, which are allocated to individuals, institutions or local areas according to principles such as need, time-related, status or economic variables.

3.5 Equity and the allocation of burdens

Long-term care creates enormous social and economic challenges to those people affected, care receivers as well as care givers. Within welfare states there is some agreement that costs of long-term care should not be left entirely to individuals in need of care and their closest relatives as principal care givers. However, opinions as to the extent to which public action should be taken and how financing responsibilities should be shared differ widely. In general, public support for long-term care is less developed than for example in health care or in public pension systems. Even in the Nordic countries, where residential care settings as well as social services are well developed, the bulk of care-giving is still provided informally within the household or within families (Hennessy 1997).

Private market solutions are playing a small role in long-term care, what is clearly shown by evidence. Reasons discussed, however, are quite controversial. (see chapter 2.3) Information problems or external effects might hinder the development of private market solutions. In the case of severe or long-lasting care needs, the costs of long-term care exceed the ability-to-pay of many of those who need care, even if savings and assets are considered. And even if the existence of market failure is doubted for long-term care, state intervention might still be strongly favoured for equity arguments (Scanlon 1992).

The debate on the present and future finance of long-term care is very much centred on the (potential) role of the public and the social insurance sector, possibilities to support private insurance solutions and the question whether or not and how to include assets in the design of financing long-term care programmes. Current developments are characterised by approaches to develop a care market and to support intermediate or mixed solutions between sectors. The role of the public sector is increasingly focused on its role as a regulator, purchaser of care and provider of cash benefits rather than the actual provider of care.

The role of the informal sector is all too often neglected. This also disregards the fact that any decision regarding public intervention in long-term care and related public policy fields – even if not directly focused on informal care – does have considerable impacts on the distribution of burdens within the informal sector. And because this is the sector where the bulk of long-term care is provided and financed, it has the most important impact on the overall distribution of burdens in the finance of long-term care.

The burdens to be shared

Analysing equity in the finance of welfare programmes usually considers taxes, social insurance contributions, private insurance contributions and out-of-pocket payments, but ignores informal non-monetary transfers (e.g. van Doorslaer, Wagstaff, Rutten 1993). An approach limited to monetary transfers in analysing equity in the finance of any welfare issue only is an adequate approach if there is a clear-cut distinction between the monetary and the non-monetary sphere and the formal and the informal sector. And it has, of course, advantages in the quantitative analysis regarding data availability, comparability and handling. A clear-cut distinction between the formal and the informal sector – at least to some extent – applies to the health care sector. However, there are important examples that even here the ignorance of informal non-monetary contributions might be problematic. For example, a tendency to further reduce the length of stay in hospitals is not just about increasing efficiency in the health sector, but also about shifting responsibilities – and costs – from the hospital sector to other professional sectors as well as to the informal sector.

Analysing equity in the finance of long-term care just based on what has been mentioned above as the traditional monetary means of financing welfare would partly describe the distribution of burdens. This, however, would certainly not be a reflection of the whole picture. As informal long-term care covers the bulk of long-term care needs and as there is no clear-cut distinction between informal and formal tasks, the distribution of informal care-giving has a most important influence on the overall distribution of the burdens of financing long-term care. Hence, the approach of this study is to recognise the role of informal care-giving as in-kind contributions in the finance of long-term care.

The first and most obvious way in which the public sector 'designs' the allocation of burdens in the finance of long-term care is through taxes and social insurance contributions. Here the state directly takes responsibility for the process of raising and collecting funds, with a variety of principles according to which burdens are distributed (see below). Depending on the extent to which levying taxes or social insurance contributions is connected to taking responsibilities in the provision of long-term care, this means an exemption of the private sector from investments regarding protection against potential future long-term care needs. However, as shown before, such investments – at least in the formal private sector – have been comparatively small, even in case of very limited public responsibilities.

Whereas social insurance contributions tend to be earmarked, this is the exception with taxes. Earmarking, however, usually just refers to a specific field of intervention, for example social insurance contributions for health care. Apart from this general rule the actual use might differ quite considerably: Variations in the distribution among competing claims such as prevention, acute care, rehabilitation, and – as far as covered by the health insurance branch – long-term care favours different individuals or groups within society.

Apart from pooling funds in the public (or closely related social insurance) sector, public bodies also might intervene in a variety of ways to establish or to strengthen private solutions in the formal as well as in the informal sector and, hence, contribute – explicitly or implicitly – to a specific distribution of burdens in the finance of long-term care.

Private insurance might occur in a range of forms from purely private insurance with no specific public intervention (apart from the general regulation of insurance markets) to compulsory insurance models, where insurance companies act in a highly regulated private sector. Such regulation might include the obligation to contract or the obligation to offer specific basic insurance packages. Private insurance solutions with considerable public intervention are in fact one of the approaches to be found in a number of proposals for the future finance of long-term care (see e.g. Scanlon 1992; Felder, Zweifel 1998).

Out-of-pocket payments occur in two distinct forms: On the one hand, out-of-pocket payments have to be made in a model of purely private consumption of goods and services. Here the state does not intervene in the finance of these goods and services. On the other hand, out-of-pocket payments occur as co-payments to goods and services offered by the public sector or financed – up to these co-payments – by private insurance companies. In one case, finance is a purely private obligation either because there is no public intervention or because individuals prefer to act in the private sector despite the fact that there is public long-term care finance. In the case of user charging, individuals have to make co-payments to receive specific goods or services – at least if they are above a given income level.

User charging has always played an important role in long-term care and tends to become generally more important in welfare. The objective of such out-of-pocket payments is either to contribute to the finance of services and/or to introduce economic incentives. Economic incentives may be designed to prevent or to reduce moral hazard, that is a tendency towards over-consumption because of the lacking price signal, or to guide allocation in a specific direction, for example, by making residential or domiciliary care economically more or less attractive.

Regarding the future finance of long-term care, debates are increasingly focusing on the potential role of assets. It is argued that elderly people, the majority of those in need of long-term care, increasingly have considerable assets that could be used as a major source for financing long-term care needs. This, however, is not a novel approach. On the contrary, social assistance schemes have been and – as far as long-term care is concerned – are still a major source of financing long-term care. In social assistance schemes means-testing often does not just refer to income but to income and assets. The reactive decision on the individual level to such regulations on the meso-level are asset transfers and estate planning to protect assets from being used for financing long-term care provision. This becomes particularly relevant in the case of care in nursing homes. The way assets are recognised in the design of public responsibilities in care does create considerable financial incentives for the behaviour and the attitudes in the private sector, which in turn forces the public sector to adapt their policy approach. (For a discussion see e.g. Walker, Burwell 1998.)

Moving from the formal to the informal sector the finance of long-term care shifts from financing through money transfers to non-monetary transfers. But, there is no clear-cut distinction between the formal and the informal sphere, and monetary and non-monetary transfers in the informal sphere. This has been shown throughout this study. The broad range of transfers within households and families can be illustrated by some basic examples: Monetary transfers might occur between family members, for example, money from family members that are not involved in the actual care-giving process to those in need of care or to those who actually offer care. Another form of monetary transfer occurs if there are payment for care programmes financed in the public sector (or in an insurance market) offering payments to care receivers or care givers. Care money to care receivers might be used to transfer money to informal care givers. Another form of compensation might occur in the form of bequests. Finally, informal care-giving is offered without direct compensation. Here, informal care-giving does not just incur considerable opportunity costs (Ettner 1996; Carmichael, Charles 1998). Furthermore, many informal care givers might – and in fact have to – finance additional costs of caring – such as travel costs, costs of special dietary requirements or costs of special aids.

Explicit legal obligations of long-term care might exist with regard to rules of allocating burdens between the formal and the informal sector. If there is neither a legal obligation to care for family members nor a public approach to secure sufficient provision of care, the provision and finance of care is left to the private formal or informal sector. Then, to what extent care is organised in the informal sector is a question of values and attitudes towards informal care-giving as well as the economic opportunities to organise alternative forms of care.

The subjects of allocating burdens

The focal units among whom the burdens in the finance of long-term care are to be shared are individuals and – as final or intermediate focal units – households, families, companies, or geographical areas. Local areas or even countries could become the focal unit if, for example, supranational organisations, such as the European Union, would raise money in order to improve territorial justice and to support long-term care initiatives in the member states accordingly.

Those who are liable to pay taxes or social insurance contributions are not necessarily identical with those who bear the burden. For example, in the case of social insurance contributions paid by employers and employees or in a private insurance model in the case of private insurance contributions, it is far from clear who finally has to bear the burden. The difference between 'statutory' incidence (the question of who actually has to pay) and 'economic' incidence (the question of who has finally to bear the burden) is determined by the design of taxes and contributions (the definition of the source to be taxed, etc.) as well as the structure of the respective markets, in particular with regard to supply and demand elasticities. (For a discussion of the concept of incidence see e.g. Musgrave 1959; Musgrave, Musgrave 1989; Blankart 1991; Cullis, Jones 1998)

This question of incidence is most important for the design and the analysis of public finance programmes and the evaluation of related distributional issues. Although there are theoretically clear answers to the incidence of taxes and social insurance contributions, considerable variations occur in empirical evidence (discussed e.g. in Atkinson, Stiglitz 1980). This is even more true for comparative research, as incidence might differ quite considerably across countries. Empirical studies on distributional effects are therefore based on incidence assumptions. For example, equity analyses in health care by van Doorslaer, Wagstaff, Rutten (1993) are based on the assumption that personal income and property taxes have to be borne by taxpayers, corporate income taxes by shareholders, sales and excise taxes by consumers, and employee and employer health insurance contributions by employees.

As mentioned before, the role of private insurance in long-term care is limited as is the financial ability of the majority of the population to pay for severe and long-lasting care needs by buying the relevant services on the formal market. Hence, without public intervention the bulk of long-term care tends to remain in the private informal sector. Here, the question of 'incidence' occurs in another form. If the costs of long-term care have to be borne in the informal sector, burdens are distributed according to features that will differ quite considerably between households and families. And they are rather difficult to quantify. Looking at the 'outcome' of this intra-family or intra-household distribution makes clear that the bulk of long-term care-giving is borne by women within families, in particular as spouses, daughters and daughters-in-law. In addition, men play a considerable role as informal care givers as retired men caring for their partner (see chapter 2.1). For all of them – and in particular for those in the working age – opportunity costs are substantial (see chapter 2.1).

The principles of allocating burdens

The most widespread explicit principle in allocating burdens in the public finance of welfare programmes are *economic variables*. Here, the term 'economic variables' will be used to point at criteria considering economic characteristics such as ability-to-pay, income, assets or consumption. Related questions are at the core of the theory of taxation and discussed extensively in the literature (see e.g. Stiglitz 2000; Musgrave, Musgrave 1989; Cullis, Jones 1998).

Financing welfare programmes through social security systems or tax systems is relating burdens to income, property or wealth. By setting specific relationships between these features and the financial burdens, systems take account of different levels of income or wealth. Although relating burdens to wealth is confronted with some problems of practicality, wealth or private savings are increasingly seen as one of the key sources for financing long-term care in the future, not necessarily as a taxable source, but as a means of private solutions to be supported by fiscal policies (Garber 1996). Apart from income and wealth, a broader concept of ability-to-pay might also consider additional variables, such as the number of dependent children in the household or special care needs from family members.

The relationship between ability-to-pay – however the concept is defined – and the actual extent to which taxes or social insurance contributions have to be paid is described by the so-called 'progressivity' of a financing system. In a progressive system payments for long-term care rise as a proportion of income as income rises, that is the economically better off have to spend a larger proportion of their income for financing long-term care. In a regressive system payments for long-term care fall as a proportion of income as income rises, whereas in a proportional system the proportion of the income that has to be spent on payments for long-term care is the same with variations in income.

Personal income tax systems are usually designed as progressive systems (at least up to a certain level of income) as the proportion of taxes that have to be paid rises with income. Social insurance contributions – in an overall perspective – tend to be regressive systems. This is because social insurance contributions tend to be proportional to income or earnings up to a specific ceiling. Above this ceiling no additional contributions have to be paid. Hence, those with higher earnings (above the ceiling) have to spend a lower proportion of their earnings on social insurance contributions than those with lower income.

Progressivity indices are a means to measure the extent of progressivity, which enables progressivity to be compared across different systems (Lambert 1989). The 'Kakwani index', as used for example in the van Doorslaer, Wagstaff, Rutten (1993) health studies, is based on the concept of the Lorenz curve. This curve describes the distribution of income among the population by plotting the cumulative proportions of the population against the cumulative proportions of income. For calculating the Kakwani index, two 'concentration curves' are compared: The Lorenz curve for pre-tax income and the tax (or social insurance contributions, etc.) concentration curve. In a progressive system the tax concentration curve lies outside the pre-tax income curve, in a perfectly proportional system they would be identical, whereas in a regressive system the tax concentration curve lies inside the pre-tax income curve. The Kakwani index then is calculated by subtracting the concentration index for tax payments from the Gini coefficient for pre-tax income. One of the problems with this and other progressivity indices is that progressivity changes over income levels. A tax or insurance system that is progressive in lower income levels but becomes regressive in higher income levels is not adequately reflected in the index. It might even result in an index pointing at proportionality of the system.

Economic principles also occur in the design of out-of-pocket payments, in particular with co-payments that have to be made in residential or domiciliary care. Apart from a basic choice whether or not to introduce co-payments, explicit economic principles in out-of-pocket payments as a source of financing long-term care occur in the definition of the concept of ability-to-pay (based on income, savings, taking account of financially restricting situations, etc.) as well as the actual relationship between ability-to-pay and the extent of co-payments to be made.

The idea of progressivity can be applied to co-payments as with taxes or insurance contributions. Flat-rate co-payments that do not take the income level or the ability-to-pay into account are regressive. The same is true for proportionate co-payments with a ceiling in absolute terms above which no additional co-payments have to be made. Here co-payments are proportionate up to that ceiling, but are overall regressive. A common solution to the design of co-payments are co-payments as a flat-rate payment for those above a specific income level, whereas those with low income are exempted. Such co-payments are progressive if just the two income groups are compared as such, but regressive within the two groups.

Apart from criteria related to a broader concept of ability-to-pay, taxes or contributions might also be related to either the consumption of individuals, or the extent to which individuals (potentially) will benefit (Stiglitz 2000). Taxing consumption vs. taxing income is related to the question whether or not and to what extent savings and the return to savings should be exempted from taxation. This might, for example, be used to create incentives for private solutions in the finance of long-term care by exempting savings from taxation that are dedicated for potential long-term care needs in old age.

A further criterion might relate taxes to the benefits individuals will receive from public services. Taxes then would be seen as 'fees' for the future provision of public services or public benefits. In the actual design, this would require a definition of the risk of each individual regarding the future need of long-term care. Apart from the difficult task of assessing individual risk regarding future health problems and long-term care needs, this tends to be challenged from equity considerations. In this respect long-term care is similar to health care, where public schemes tend to be financed according to ability-to-pay whereas the actual provision is oriented to health needs. *Risk* is commonly not seen as an adequate or desirable principle in the allocation of burdens with regard to basic health needs and with regard to health problems arising from factors beyond individuals' responsibility. There are, however, debates on how to treat those health problems which arise because of choices freely made by individuals (see e.g. Le Grand 1991).

As in the provision of care, *status variables* tend to be used as additional principles in the finance of care in a variety of ways. In many social insurance systems occupational status becomes an additional principle of allocating burdens if contributions differ across occupational sections of the insurance system. If a person has to be cared for in a nursing home or by social services, the degree of relationship might be used as an additional principle for allocating burdens by obliging children, partners or other family members to (partly) finance these services. Residents in a specific local area might have to make lower co-payments than non-residents in institutional care settings, or national citizens are exempted from co-payments whereas non-citizens are not. In all these examples, *mixed principles* are used to allocate burdens.

As long as the burdens to be shared are easily measured in monetary terms and the allocation principle is clearly defined, there is not much room for *'implicit principles'*, as it is the case with income taxes or social insurance contributions. Implicit principles, however, become increasingly important if the finance of long-term care is organised in the private sector with a regulatory role of public bodies. In a compulsory private insurance scheme, information and informal connections, as well as health status might become implicit principles in allocating burdens. The level of information becomes increasingly important if there is a broad diversity of insurance contracts offered in the private sector, if the use of informal connections might help to get access to financially more attractive insurance contracts or if selection according to health status might occur. The extent to which these implicit principles determine the burden of financing long-term care depends on whether or not and how the private insurance sector is regulated.

Other implicit principles come into operation if families are explicitly obliged to care for close relatives, or if the public role is of subsidiary nature. As for economic reasons, formal private solutions tend to be rather limited, the actual distribution of the burdens lies to a considerable extent within the private informal sphere. The decision-making process within families depends on a number of issues, such as values and attitudes towards informal care-giving, gender roles in society, as well as incentives created by the economic environment or welfare state programmes. Incentives set by the public sector to offer informal care-giving include payments for care, the recognition of informal care-giving in social security programmes as well as the creation of full- or part-time leave programmes. On the other hand, public programmes might include restricting incentives regarding the provision of informal care. Welfare benefits with a strong labour market link may have this effect as well as an economic and social environment that requires two incomes to 'finance' a family. These approaches represent different equity choices, not just with regard to the distribution of long-term care obligations. Their focus – and often their primary focus – is on the distribution of welfare benefits, the distribution of formal and informal work, etc.

Table 3.3 Choices in the finance of long-term care

WHAT (burdens)	burdens *by means of* contributions in cash / in-kind regulation
WHOM (subjects)	individuals families / households institutions geographical areas
HOW (principles)	income wealth ability-to-pay egalitarian benefits risk status mixed implicit

The interpretations of equity in the finance of long-term care are summarised in Table 3.3. Methods used in social and fiscal policy to achieve an equitable distribution of these burdens are regulation, cash contributions (imposing taxes or social insurance payments and regulating private insurance contributions or out-of-pocket payments) as well as regulating in-kind contributions, with economic, status and implicit principles as the guiding rules of allocating these burdens.

3.6 Conclusions

Research on equity issues in welfare state policies has concentrated on different approaches. On the one hand, there is the normative approach of how equity ought to be defined in social policy or in specific social policy fields. On the other hand, empirical research is aimed at studying social justice judgements or at studying distributional outcomes and testing specific interpretations of equity. These studies are asking, for example, to what extent the consumption of health care services is related to a specific interpretation of need, whether there is discrimination in the take-up of specific services regarding age, sex, occupational status, etc. or whether taxes and social insurance contributions to finance the welfare state are related to income or a broader concept of ability-to-pay. The fact that many of these studies show considerable 'inequities' is not just because of some external factors that policies did not succeed to produce a more 'equitable' distribution, but because actual equity choices were not designed in a way that this could lead to the respective 'ideal' distribution against which real outcomes are analysed.

In addition, even if there is public intervention in a specific social policy field, equity choices do not necessarily include explicit decisions regarding who will receive what share of the resource, and who has to bear what share of the burden. To a considerable extent, public choices just create boundaries and leave further operationalisation to other actors in the respective field.

An approach recognising that there is no single equity interpretation in actual social policies – not even in single social policy fields – is widely missing. Long-term care is a prime example for such a policy context. There will be some agreement that support ought to be shared according to need, and burdens according to ability-to-pay. Whether to cover needs through services or cash benefits, to what extent to provide care in the formal sector, or how to divide responsibilities between the private (formal and/or informal) and the public sector are just three examples for variations, which make it a most interesting case for the use of the concept of equity choices.

The approach of equity choices as an analytical tool allows a systematic analysis of equity as it is approached in welfare state design. This approach does not start from any normative approach how equity should be defined nor from a more colloquial interpretation of equity. In contrast to these approaches it recognises the complexity of equity interpretations that are found in any single policy field. The three elements, brought together, create a wide range of potential equity interpretations. Hence, the approach of equity choices offers an important addition to existing research strands.

In this study the framework is applied to long-term care systems in four European countries. The analytical framework, though, offers an effective tool going beyond this research question. The framework might as well be used in other social policy fields, in comparative perspective as well as in single country or even smaller scale units, it might be used to focus on specific actors designing equity choices or those affected by such choices.

The tool might be used for the analysis of similarities and differences, causal factors for specific choices or the consequences of equity choices.

4 Investigating Long-Term Care Policies in Europe

The objective of parts four and five of the study is to comparatively analyse how different countries approach the objective of equity in long-term care through choices in the allocation of resources and burdens. Part four proceeds as follows: The analysis is introduced by a general discussion of the comparative approach in social policies. (chapter 4.1) First of all, the objectives of comparative social research in social policy and the utilised approaches will be examined. Then, following the objectives of this study, the countries for the empirical analysis will be selected: Austria, Italy, the Netherlands and the United Kingdom. The chapter concludes with an investigation of possibilities and constraints of cross-national comparative research with special respect to issues arising in the comparative analysis of long-term care.

Chapter 4.2 introduces equity as a welfare state objective. The study proceeds by using a set of such objectives underlying the concept of modern welfare states to investigate whether or not and to what extent actual equity choices in different countries contribute to the achievement of these objectives. The chapter also includes an overview of various approaches to categorise welfare states. Underlying concepts offer additional information on implicit ideas about equity. They are, however, limited as a tool or as a framework against which equity choices could be investigated.

Then, chapter 4.3 presents an overview to long-term care in Europe and, in more detail, information on the design of the long-term care systems in the four countries selected. For all these countries key figures describing the long-term care system as well as the social and economic care environment will be presented alongside basic information on residential care, domiciliary care, payments for care to care receivers, payments for care to informal care givers, informal care, and the finance of care in the four countries.

4.1 Cross-country comparative analysis in long-term care

Ideas and approaches of comparative analysis

Comparative research, in the sense of cross-country comparative research, is interested in analysing similarities and differences across countries. Other terms used in this context, such as cross-national, cross-cultural, cross-societal, trans-cultural or trans-national studies, might point at a specific interest in the comparative analysis, however, usage of this terminology is not homogeneous (Øyen 1990). For an introduction to comparative social research in social policy see e.g. Jones (1985), Clasen (1999), Hantrais, Mangen (1996), Janoski, Hicks (1994a), Øyen (1990), or Ragin (1987) and – with respect to specific features in long-term care – Tester (1999).

The objective of cross-country comparative research is to search for and to find rules or generalisations in the respective countries, cultures or societies regarding similarities and differences in specific characteristics and features. The interest, however, is not just in investigating similarities and differences. Comparative research helps to escape cultural hegemony, to learn about other societies and cultures and to learn more about the own society and culture and to improve ex-post as well as ex-ante analysis in social policy (Jones 1985; Janoski, Hicks 1994b).

Four basic types of studies can be distinguished when regarding the role of the countries in the analysis: The countries to be studied might be the object of the study (the main interest lies in the countries studied), the context of the study (testing research results in various countries), the unit of the analysis (relating specific features to the characteristic of a country), or countries can be put in a trans-national context regarding countries as part of the international system (Kohn 1989).

In the comparative analysis of social policy issues at least three basic approaches can be identified (Jones 1985; Hauser 1991; Higgins 1987). In the *institutional approach* the focus is on the (institutional) system of social protection in the countries to be studied. In a second approach, the situation of a group of individuals, characterised by specific features, is the focus of the study (*social groups approach*). This approach is followed in the comparative analysis of specific socio-economic groups such as the poor, children, women, or the elderly. Finally, an approach focusing on a specific problem can be identified (*social problems approach*). Here, the analysis follows an issue that is identified as a social policy or welfare state issue, such as discrimination, poverty or illness. In reality, a combination of these approaches will occur. For example, this study – analysing equity choices in long-term care policies – follows the question of how welfare states deal with a specific problem by establishing or promoting specific settings, 'institutionalising' explicit or implicit choices regarding the allocation of resources and burdens.

As for the development of comparative research, it has been dominated for a long time by either historical comparative research or comparative research based on quantitative aggregate data. Studies either tend to look at inputs (e.g. social expenditure, the type of benefits) or at outputs (e.g. income distribution before and after welfare benefits). A prominent example for the first type is Wilensky (1975) analysing social expenditure. Others spend more attention at the content of the welfare state, that is specific characteristics. An early example for this approach is Titmuss (1958) or more recently Esping-Andersen (1990). And there is growing literature on analysing outputs (rather than the broader concept of outcome) of the welfare state, in particular in research on income distribution and poverty (e.g. Smeeding, O'Higgins, Rainwater 1989), and increasingly in other fields of social policy such as health (e.g. van Doorslaer, Wagstaff, Rutten 1993).

Regarding the dualism of quantitative and qualitative comparative research, quantitative analysis clearly dominates the research agenda. Although there have been considerable improvements in the availability of data across countries, there is still a considerable lack of comparable data in many areas. And long-term care is a prime example of this problem as will be shown below. This among other things contributes to a concentration of research questions on issues such as the analysis of aggregate budget information or the analysis of cash benefits, whereas other issues remain underinvestigated. Examples are the analysis of in-kind benefits, the outcome of the welfare state (unlike the output) or the process between inputs and outputs. With regard to long-term care, the neglect or underestimation of gender issues and the role of social services in 'mainstream' comparative research is very important. Only more recent research has emphasised these issues as important elements for the comparative understanding of welfare states (e.g. Alber 1995, Anttonen, Sipilä 1996, Knijn, Kremer 1997). Lacks in comparative welfare state research are increasingly recognised and have also lead to a 're-discovery' of qualitative research (e.g. Hantrais, Mangen 1996) as well as attempts to combine qualitative and quantitative approaches (e.g. Ragin 1987).

Parallel to the public interest in long-term care issues, comparative research in long-term care is relatively new on the research agenda. However, as briefly shown in the introduction there is a growing number of studies. Most recent examples are Pacolet, Bouten, Lanoye, Versieck

(1999a) who are analysing social protection for dependency in old age, Tester (1996) who is studying origins, substance and outcome in community care in six countries, Weekers, Pijl (1998) and Hutten, Kerkstra (1996) who are analysing home care and social services, Weekers, Pijl (1998) and Evers, Pijl, Ungerson (1994), as well as Glendinning, McLaughlin (1993) who are studying payments for care or Rostgaard, Fridberg (1998) who are studying the systems of care for children and elderly people in seven European countries. Many of the existing studies do include detailed information on the institutional and policy mix in the countries under investigation, offering a most important source for any further comparative research.

Comparing equity choices in long-term care

The objective of the empirical part of this study is to comparatively analyse equity choices and to contrast them with equity objectives. The position of this study in the comparative analysis of long-term care systems is shown in Figure 4.1. The focus is on the characteristics of 'equity choices' as designed in welfare state programmes to regulate, to finance and/or to deliver long-term care and the consequences with regard to the achievement of basic equity objectives. The conceptual issues with regard to these factors have been introduced and discussed in parts 2 and 3.

Extending such an analysis from the single-country perspective to a comparative cross-country analysis adds some constraints (see below), but at the same time increases its potential in a number of ways. It creates or at least enhances the opportunity to study variations and similarities in policy design by investigating alternative approaches. This becomes even more important as long-term care is characterised by a broad mix of alternatives in terms of public vs. private responsibilities, formal vs. informal care, paid vs. unpaid care, cash vs. in-kind benefits or the mix in the institutional settings. This makes long-term care a most interesting case for shifting boundaries in the design of social policies. And it is important as welfare and social policy 'regimes' are confronted with the implications of increasingly globalised markets and communications.

Selecting the case-studies

The selection of countries to be analysed can be oriented at two distinct approaches: selecting 'most similar cases' vs. selecting 'diverse cases' or the method of agreement vs. the method of difference (Janoski, Hicks 1994b). Whereas the choice of most similar cases allows the researcher to more clearly identify differences in specific variables and to explain specific variations, such a choice narrows the range of variations in variables and potential causal relationships.

Figure 4.1 Foci in comparing equity choices in long-term care systems

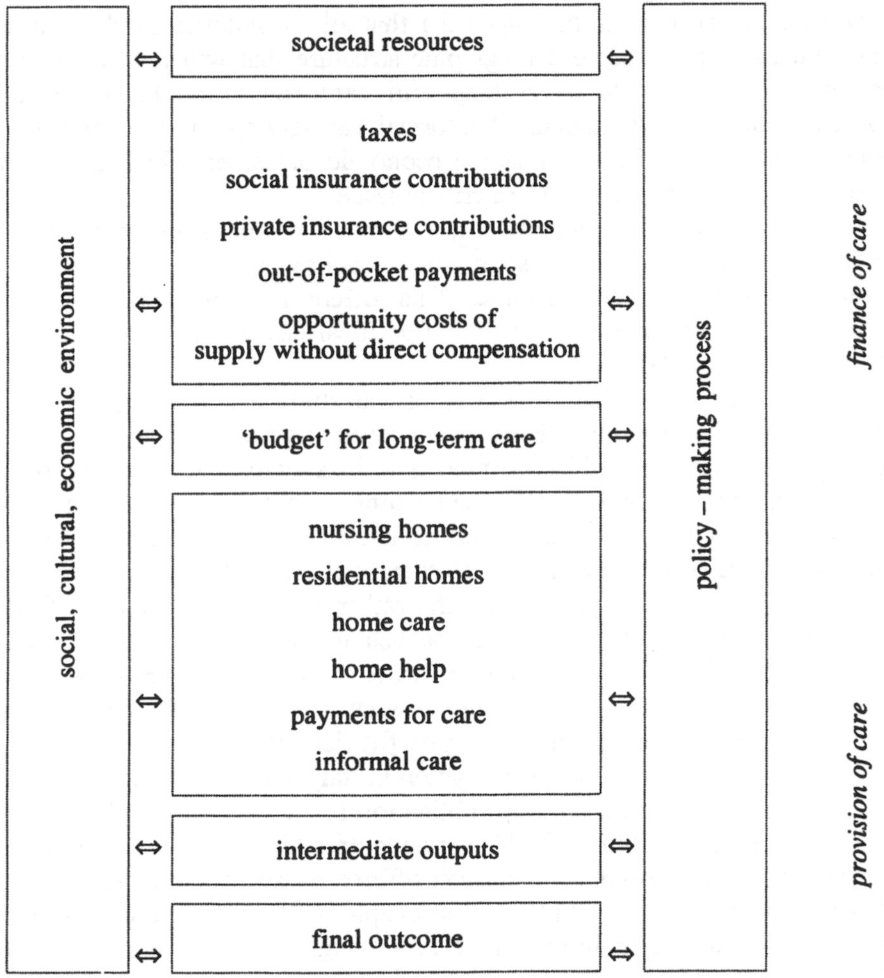

A combination of the two approaches seems most adequate for the research question of this study. Public intervention in long-term care is rather restricted in less industrialised countries, and even in many industrialised countries public long-term care intervention occurs at a later stage in the development of the welfare state. Apart from choosing countries that have developed a certain level of state intervention in long-term care, the outcome of the study will be more significant if these countries have to act in a similar cultural, social, political and economic environment (Hauser 1991). This is the case for the member states of the European Union. Apart from the similarities in their political and cultural background, they also share major demographic, social and economic challenges. It has been described in more detail in chapter 2.1 that all the industrialised countries face changes in the socio-demographic structure that will tend to require additional resources to cover long-term care needs and to reduce the potential quantitative amount of informal care-giving. At the same time these countries realise considerable economic pressures which makes an expansion of social expenditure a critical issue.

Though economic integration has shown enormous progress in the European Union, differences in social policy and in welfare state conceptions remain considerable. This offers an interesting case for studying diversity in an economic and political environment characterised by increasing similarities.

The countries selected for the empirical study are Austria, Italy, the Netherlands, and the United Kingdom. These countries share similarities in their political and cultural background as well as major demographic, social and economic challenges. At the same time – as will be shown in more detail in chapter 4.2 – the four countries represent quite different approaches regarding the design of their welfare state. As explicit and clear-cut welfare state objectives are rather rare, the selection of the countries is based on various approaches to categorise welfare states. Closely related to the long-term care issue, the four countries show quite important differences regarding legal regulations of the division between family and public responsibilities in care (Millar, Warman 1996). Whereas there exists an extended family obligation in Italy and to a smaller extent in Austria, there is no clear-cut legal obligation in the United Kingdom and a clear state responsibility in the Netherlands. In addition, the four countries fit with different welfare state clusters offered by authors such as Esping-Andersen (1990) or Ferrera (1993) (see chapter 4.2). As with regard to data availability and comparability, this selection might create some restrictions. However, by restricting the possibility of quantitative analysis it offers an opportunity to analyse a broader diversity of equity choices and herewith gives a better picture of how different countries deal with long-term care issues against rather similar demographic, political and economic circumstances.

Possibilities and constraints in the comparative analysis

Comparative social research in general is faced with a number of issues that might create considerable additional difficulties that do not occur (or at least do not occur to the same extent) in the analysis of a single country or region. These potential restrictions include problems and constraints arising from definitions and concepts as well as with data availability and comparability. An additional challenge arises from language differences. As will be shown here, these issues tend to be even more severe in studying long-term care (Tester 1999; Sipilä 1997; Edvartsen 1996; Doty 1988). As Jones (1985) described it: '... personal social care happens to be one of the least researched and least documented areas for comparative study. This neglect of what represents, after all, the oldest form of social intervention may seem ironic yet is understandable, none the less. It represents a messy area for research.'

First of all, problems and constraints arise from differences in definitions, a lack of conceptual consistency, and differences in long-term care practice. Analysing long-term care issues, hence, requires a clear concept of what long-term care is and how the target population can be defined. The three main approaches for such a definition – measuring impairments, measuring the inability or the limitations in fulfilling certain activities, and measuring the amount of help needed – have been briefly described in chapter 2.2. But there is no generally accepted definition that allows for a clear and objectively observable categorisation. In practice, very different approaches are applied and room for discretion in the assessment often plays an important role.

Variations also arise from the design of long-term care systems. The division of public and private as well as formal and informal responsibilities often is vaguely defined. For example, social services may be based on very different concepts regarding tasks and professional requirements. Very different standards are used with regard to the tasks of home nursing and home help. The dividing line between nursing homes and residential homes is often not found between single homes but within one home, apart from the fact that such a clear dividing line is not necessarily desirable. In general, there are no clear-cut basic institutions. And finally, there are variations in the labels used to describe specific institutions or services. The same terminology might be used to describe different services and different labels might be used to describe similar services. Often, this is even true within countries. A number of examples are presented in Kerkstra, Hutten (1996).

The second bulk of problems arises from data availability and comparability. The reason for the considerable lack of data in quantitative and qualitative terms is at least threefold: limited public responsibility and awareness of the issue, the complexity of long-term care, and the rather decentralised decision-making and data-gathering processes.

Relevant data is to be found under different headings, such as in health, elderly, family, or invalidity categories, but there is no specific long-term care category (for example in the Eurostat classification). Generally, it is just a by-product and does not give a full picture of the issue, apart from the fact that the boundaries between, for example, social care and health care are not clear-cut. As mentioned above, this lack of clear-cut definitions and labelling also applies to institutions and services within long-term care. As a result, we miss systematic data-collections for long-term care, all too often even within countries as well.

Existing datasets, such as the European Community Household Panel (ECHP) or the Socio-Economic Panel (SOEP) in Germany, do include a number of variables for the study of long-term care issues. The number of relevant observations in panel data is, however, usually rather small. This becomes even more problematic as enormous variations in long-term care systems within countries require a breakdown by local areas. For example, in the SOEP 1985-1991, the number of disabled people (all age groups) is between 126 and 176 (Edvartsen 1996). Many datasets do not cover people cared for in residential care settings, an important group for the study of long-term care issues in terms of the extent of care needs as well as the cost of care.

The diversity of data may be illustrated by another example: The Austrian attendance allowance is paid to 4.0% of the Austrian population. About three quarters of the beneficiairies are 75 years of age or older. In the Austrian ECHP data 6.7% are reported as 'severely hampered in daily activities' (Heitzmann 1999). Only half of them are 65 years of age or older. The attendance allowance is given on the basis of a medical certificate assessing care needs (for more details see chapter 4.2). ECHP data is based on self-reported inabilities or limitations. Whereas in the attendance allowance scheme there is no age limit, ECHP covers those 15 years of age and older. Those living in institutions are included in the attendance allowance programme, but not in the ECHP data. Altogether, these data discrepancies make comparison even more problematic.

A further problem in cross-country comparative research which is often ignored arises from language. In the context of care this is discussed by Ungerson (1990). The issue of language in comparative research includes the understanding and meaning of terms in a cultural context, the translation in the process of collecting and analysing data as well as the issue of publication in one language, where potential readers come into play.

Pointing out these difficulties in comparative research, in particular in long-term care, should make research and the use of research more sensitive for possibilities and constraints in comparative research. The best way to deal with the problems is to clarify the approaches used in research with regard to their outcome and their potential shortcomings.

4.2 Objectives, regimes and choices

This study attempts to investigate equity choices as introduced conceptually in part 3 with regard to basic equity objectives in welfare states. There is broad agreement on the importance of equity as an objective in the welfare state. Very rarely, however, is this objective made more explicit. Other than with, for example, efficiency, there is no clear-cut single definition of equity that would find broad support across countries and across various fields of welfare and that, at the same time, would allow a systematic evaluation of respective equity choices to achieve that objective.

This study proposes a set of equity objectives. These objectives will be discussed in more detail in this chapter. They are to be found in different combinations and given different weight in various welfare states. Therefore, this chapter starts with an overview of various approaches to categorise welfare states. These efforts are based on different features in the design, the process and the outcome of welfare states aiming at types, regimes or families of welfare states. As will be shown, most of these efforts are aimed at a cross-sectional categorisation that gives a broad picture of such families. They are, however, limited with regard to specific policy areas, as has been shown repeatedly for long-term care (see e.g. Anttonen, Sipilä 1996; Tester 1999). Commenting on welfare state regimes, therefore, will be used to discuss various ideas about the welfare state and, hence, to inform the set of equity objectives that will be used as the reference point to investigate equity choices to be found in European long-term care systems.

Welfare state regimes

For at least 40 years the analysis of welfare states and the development of welfare state models – whether they are called models, clusters, regimes, or families, etc. – has made up a major part in comparative research in social policy. Wilensky, Lebeaux (1958) distinguishing between residual and institutional welfare state models and Titmuss (1958) analysing the industrial achievement-performance model and the institutional-redistributive model are important early representatives of this research tradition. They have considerably influenced the following works by researchers such as Mishra (1981) who distinguishes between residual, institutional and socialist models. Whereas in early conceptualisations models often represented stages in the development of welfare states, research then moved on to analyse specific characteristics of different models, not representing a stage in the process of the development of another welfare state model but distinct approaches to welfare and the welfare state.

Most recently Esping-Andersen's (1990) distinction between liberal, corporatist, and social democratic welfare states (see Table 4.1) introduced a new wave of debate regarding welfare state classification. At the core of his approach are two distinct features: de-commodification which requires that 'citizens can freely, and without potential loss of job, income, or general welfare, opt out of work when they themselves consider it necessary' (Esping-Andersen 1990: 23), and stratification which points at the role of the state as 'an active force in the ordering of social relations' (Esping-Andersen 1990: 23).

Table 4.1 Welfare state clusters according to Esping-Andersen

Welfare state cluster	*represented by ...*
Liberal welfare states	Australia, Canada, Switzerland, United States, (*United Kingdom*)
Corporatist welfare states	*Austria*, Belgium, France, Germany, *Italy*
Social-democratic welfare states	Denmark, Finland, *Netherlands*, Norway, Sweden

Source: Esping-Andersen (1990)

With regard to welfare states promoting equity and equality concerns, liberal welfare states are characterised by a residual safety net for the poor, social-democratic welfare regimes by universalist benefits and vertical redistribution, whereas corporatist welfare states are typified by benefits following occupational segregation.

The classification of welfare states by Esping-Andersen has opened a wide debate on methodological issues of comparing welfare states (see e.g. subsequent references or Spicker 1996; Kohl 1993). It has created an incentive for further approaches to classify welfare states, either following in the steps of Esping-Andersen or using different approaches in classifying welfare states (e.g. Ferrera 1993; Leibfried 1993; Lewis 1992; Bonoli 1997).

The classification by Ferrera (1993) uses coverage of social protection schemes as the main criterion for classifying welfare states. In this classification, universal welfare states and occupational welfare states are distinguished. Within the two categories a distinction is made between those countries that can be seen as either pure or mixed representatives of these two clusters. Different from other approaches to classify welfare states, Ferrera's approach is not based on a quantification of welfare benefits but on identifying characteristics of the type of social protection. This leads to a classification of welfare states (see Table 4.2) that is quite distinct from that of Esping-Andersen presented above.

Table 4.2 Welfare state clusters according to Ferrera

Welfare state cluster	*represented by ....*
Pure occupational welfare states	*Austria*, Belgium, France, Germany
Mixed occupational welfare states	*Italy*, *Netherlands*, Switzerland
Mixed universalist welfare states	Canada, New Zealand, *United Kingdom*
Pure universalist welfare states	Denmark, Finland, Norway, Sweden

Source: Ferrera (1993)

Another issue in the recent welfare state debate is the question about the existence of further welfare state models such as the southern European welfare model. Whereas in Leibfried (1993) southern European welfare states are described as 'rudimentary welfare states' in the catching up process with limited rights to welfare, others identify the specific characteristics of the 'southern model' of welfare (e.g. Ferrera 1996; Rhodes 1997). Hard facts regarding consistent 'models' of welfare states seem rather limited which led Castles (1993) to propose 'families' of welfare states sharing common features.

Looking at issues not covered in the development of the respective models or looking in more detail at some of the issues used as criteria for classification might give a very different picture of the respective welfare state and the clustering of these states. Changing criteria for the clustering process or the weight that is given to specific criteria, might produce quite different results. This is illustrated by the discussion of how to classify Australia or the United Kingdom (Esping-Andersen 1990) as well as by the different outcomes of different approaches to welfare state classification as by Esping-Andersen's more quantitative approach (1990) and Ferrera's approach (1993) based on the type rather than the level of social protection.

Hence, welfare state models have to be seen as what they are defined, that is as models or clusters – based on a bundle of specific criteria – giving a broad picture of how welfare and welfare states are designed or what the implications in the respective countries are.

Two issues of great relevance for long-term care tend to be neglected in approaches to welfare state classification, that is the role of social services and the role of women in the care sector. As for social services, Alber (1995) or Anttonen, Sipilä (1996) recently proposed frameworks for the comparative study of social services and classification according to the organisation of social services. In order to recognise the specific features of social services Alber (1995) suggests use of the regulatory structure, the financing structure, the delivery structure and the degree of consumer power as explanatory factors in the comparative analysis of social services. Anttonen, Sipilä (1996) in their study on social care services in Europe identify social care regimes according to the options given to care receivers and care givers. These care regimes are not just characterised by the level of such options, but additionally by partly quite distinct patterns in the design of services for children and services for the elderly in a number of countries.

A lack of analysing social policy benefits and services with regard to gender implications and a limited consideration of state-family relationships (compared to the attention paid to labour markets) is one of the major criticisms with 'mainstream' welfare state classifications from a gender perspective. Following this critique various attempts have been made to recognise these issues in welfare state research (Daly 2000; Knijn, Kremer 1997; Sainsbury 1996; Daly 1994; Orloff 1993; O'Connor 1993; Lewis 1992; Langan, Ostner 1991). For example, Lewis (1992) compares welfare states on the basis whether or not and to what extent welfare states recognise women as wives and mothers and/or as workers, and proposes a categorisation of European welfare states according to strong, moderate or weak breadwinner models. The concept of 'personal autonomy' (Orloff 1993; O'Connor 1993) brings care-giving and the choices available (or not available) to care givers to the core of these discussions. Knijn, Kremer (1997: 354) emphasise the '... citizenship right to time for care and the right to professional care' as an important element for inclusive degendered citizenship.

A more specific approach of categorising welfare states is to differentiate states according to the division of private and public responsibilities. The legal obligation to care for dependent family members (other than parenting) in 16 European countries (the European Union countries plus Norway) has been analysed by Millar, Warman (1996). In their study they define four different clusters: legal obligations between extended family, legal obligations between parents and children, no clear state responsibility, and clear state responsibility. (see Table 4.3)

Table 4.3 Legal obligations to care between family members

Family / state responsibility to care between family members	*represented by ...*
Legal obligation between extended family	*Italy*, Portugal, Spain
Legal obligation between parents and children	*Austria*, Belgium, France, Germany, Greece, Luxembourg
No clear state responsibility	Ireland, *United Kingdom*
Clear state responsibility	Denmark, Finland, *Netherlands*, Norway, Sweden

Source: Millar, Warman (1996)

Italy, Portugal and Spain represent those countries with an extended family obligation to care for each other or to support each other economically. That is, in these countries public support is based on testing to what extent kin is available to support family members. This is also true for countries like Austria, Germany, France or Greece. However, in these countries family obligations are restricted to a narrower concept of family including spouses and children. In addition, increasingly, differences occur in the extent to which these obligations are enforced as new schemes of support evolved (in particular payment for care programmes) and as the perception of long-term care as a public or as a private obligation might differ quite considerably from the legal obligation.

The third group is represented by Ireland and the United Kingdom. In these countries there is no legal obligation to care for close relatives or to support them with economic means. Other than in the two groups just described, long-term care is more widely seen as a public responsibility. At the same time state responsibility is not clearly defined in these countries. In the actual design of long-term care policies family obligations occur on a discretionary level. The fourth group of clear state responsibility is represented by the Nordic countries and – although less explicit – in the Netherlands. Although there is a considerable amount of family support in these countries there is a clear public obligation to support citizens in need of care.

The fact that even in the Nordic countries it is the informal sector that offers the bulk of care-giving (see chapter 2.1) contradicts to some extent such a clear-cut distinction between the countries. Nevertheless, it might be expected that equity choices in public long-term care policies are quite distinct in countries representing the four clusters.

Equity as a welfare state objective

Approaches to define welfare states or to define social policy are manifold (see e.g. Barr 1998; Badelt, Österle 2001a; Schmidt 1998; Prisching 1996; Spicker 1995; Wilson, Wilson 1991; Schulz-Nieswandt 1991). There is broad consent regarding specific modes of state intervention being an expression of the welfare state, the boundaries however are not at all well defined. The same is true for the objectives of the welfare state. What all welfare states have in common is an – explicit or implicit – concern with the objective of equity. Equity is even at the core of welfare state and social policy objectives. Apart from this basic agreement on declaring equity as an objective, however, there is not much consensus on more precise specifications of the objective of equity.

Generally, equity objectives are objectives in terms of a fair distribution of resources and burdens. As has been emphasised earlier such a distribution includes economic as well as social aspects suggesting a set of equity objectives covering both these aspects. Starting from various pragmatic approaches to set up welfare state objectives – and there are not too many such attempts (exceptions are Goodin, Headey, Muffels, Dirven 1999; Barr 1998; Wilson, Wilson 1991 or Sanmann 1973) – at least four sets of equity objectives can be identified:

- Guaranteeing minimum standards: reduction and/or prevention of absolute poverty and/or disadvantages
- Supporting living standards: prevention of large drops in living standards
- Reducing inequality: reduction and/or prevention of relative poverty and/or disadvantages
- Promoting social integration: reduction and/or prevention of social exclusion

These objectives shall be discussed in some more detail below including the 'ideal' design of welfare state measures to achieve these objectives. It has of course to be recognised that none of these objectives exists as a single objective in any welfare state. Welfare states might emphasise one or another objective and follow and reflect one or another ideal type of a welfare state model, they do, however, deviate from these ideal types in various ways as will be shown for long-term care later on in this study.

Three objectives address quantitative dimensions, but they are not just referring to the monetary dimension of income and wealth. Poverty and/or disadvantages may also occur in 'resources' such as the availability of health services, the availability of educational opportunities, as well as such features as health status or education. The fourth objective includes a qualitative perspective relating the resource approach to the social and cultural context according to which specific resources may have different meanings for different individuals and societies.

According to the objective of reducing or preventing absolute poverty and/or disadvantages, individuals or groups should not fall under a specific minimum standard of living. Following this principle, welfare state intervention occurs when the resources of the person in need (and in fact often including that of close family members) are not sufficient to cover these needs. To what point resources of individuals or their families are taken into account, is a question of the design of welfare state policies. In long-term care practice, minimum standards occur in systems supporting the poorest or the most severely disabled who are at risk to become absolutely poor. Strict means-testing is a key characteristic of liberal or residual welfare state models. Choosing cash or in-kind benefits, the degree of the minimum standard to be defined as well as further potential elements in the design would follow additional objectives and make real welfare states deviating respectively from this ideal type.

The objective of supporting living standards is related to unpredictable or predictable drops in individual living standards. Welfare state policies following this objective are concerned with potential changes in individual situations arising from risks such as unemployment, health problems, long-term care needs, etc. A standard response of the welfare state to prevent drops in the living standard are welfare benefits following the insurance principle, that is paying contributions in order to receive benefits in case the insured event occurs. This, however, tends to require social or compulsory insurance, as otherwise coverage could not be guaranteed. In addition, by socialising certain risks it is possible to reduce risk-orientation in the design of the contributions to be paid and to recognise differences in the ability-to-pay. This kind of insurance principle is a major characteristic of corporatist ideal type welfare states. As for long-term care provision, the allocation of benefits (either cash or in-kind) would follow two main principles: the recognition of needs and the recognition of pre-benefit-income. With respect to the recognition of needs, the objective to prevent drops in the living standard is linked to the objective of horizontal equity (see below). Relating benefits to pre-benefit income would – for example – require that co-payments are designed proportionately.

Finally, equity concerns with regard to economic features might be aimed at the reduction and/or prevention of inequality. Whereas in the case of supporting living standards situations of an individual before and after the occurrence of the respective event are compared, reducing and/or preventing inequality relates the individual situation to average situations or standards in society. Depending on which groups or individuals in society are compared, vertical and horizontal (in)equality or (in)equity are distinguished. Vertical equity refers to the distribution of resources and burdens according to income, ability-to-pay or economic well-being. Promoting vertical equality requires redistribution between individuals or groups of individuals on different levels in terms of income, ability-to-pay or economic well-being. Which of these features should be used and how the respective features should be defined in the actual design of welfare benefits and their finance leaves much room for controversies (Stiglitz 2000). Horizontal equity refers to specific factors that are regarded as relevant for specific policy fields, for example health status in health care systems or age in pension systems. The relevant facts might, however, be highly controversial. There certainly is not much debate with regard to differentiation in a health care or long-term care system according to health status. Other factors such as age, family size or (former) employment status can be found in health and long-term care systems. For example, in many social insurance systems, contributions vary according to employment status. Or, benefits in long-term care systems differ according to age. Whether such factors as employment status, age, or the number of dependants should be recognised with regard to concerns of horizontal equity in care is highly debatable and many will regard them as irrelevant.

Reducing vertical inequalities is at the core of egalitarian welfare states. For the finance of long-term care this requires a progressive system. With regard to provision, long-term care resembles health care in that it primarily focuses on ideas of horizontal equality. Resources are allocated to those who are ill or in need of long-term care. In this respect policy measures are in line with the objective of supporting living standards described before. But they will differ, for example, if there is any form of user charging. Whereas supporting the objective of relative equality requires relatively higher co-payments from those with higher income, supporting the objective of preventing drops in individual living standards would require proportionate co-payments.

The objectives discussed above are dealing with the position of an individual in society regarding resources. Assistance should be aimed at those who are absolutely or relatively short of resources, and therefore unable to satisfy specific needs or at least at a lower level as other members of society. This does not necessarily touch upon the broader quality of assistance, which might be an objective of the welfare state in its own right. Long-term care is not only about income and wealth, it is not only about a certain amount of care to be delivered, but also about social integration. Here the welfare state is concerned about reduction or prevention of social exclusion and stigmatisation. Benefits should enable recipients to fully participate in social life, which includes issues such as choice, solidarity, independent living or personal autonomy.

In the 1990s the concept of social exclusion has been increasingly used alongside the concept of poverty to point to a major social policy concern, these being underlined by a range of activities and publications by the European Commission and a European Observatory on policies to combat social exclusion (see e.g. Room 1993). Various attempts have been made to define social exclusion and social inclusion and to establish the main features of this concept (see e.g. Byrne 1999; Badelt 1999; Room 1995; Rodgers, Gore, Figueiredo 1995; Jordan 1996). Whereas poverty is focusing on a lack of resources enabling individuals to participate in society, social exclusion is focused on the actual participation in society, that is on social inclusion or social integration. Income or other material resources are just one possible factor that might affect the extent of social participation. Following Commins (cit. in Badelt 1999) social participation is shaped by aspects in four different spheres. It requires an integration in the legal and civic system in a society, by, for example, establishing equal human rights for every citizen. It requires economic integration, that is having resources at disposal, for example, through the opportunity to participate in the labour market. Further, social participation requires social integration by having access to collective goods such as social services or collective infrastructure. And finally, social participation requires interpersonal integration, that is having the opportunity to establish and to cultivate relationships in smaller social networks such as families, friends, or neighbours.

Definition and even more so measurement of social integration tends to be a much more difficult task than with quantitative objectives considered before. This has to do with the 'quality' of social integration which can not be allocated like money or in-kind resources. But, there is potential to design the allocation of resources and burdens promoting specific aspects of social integration. In this respect, debates on social integration are arranged around terms such as autonomy, rights, responsibilities, solidarity, dignity, independence, etc. It is difficult, if not impossible, to draw sharp lines between the various concepts. For the purpose of this study and with regard to equity concerns two issues shall be considered: autonomy and social rights and responsibilities, incorporating the various issues mentioned before.

Autonomy is about whether people are in a position to choose freely among what they want to do and what they don't want to do. This tends to be seen as just an objective emphasising individual freedom against obligations to others. As 'positive autonomy' it does however require that people's opportunities to live an autonomous life, and hence choice, are enhanced (see e.g. Wilmot 1997). With regard to those in need of care this has been particularly strong in the 'independent living' movement. More recently, 'personal autonomy' has been a major reference point for discussing the role of informal care-giving offered within families and the division of informal unpaid care between men and women (see e.g. O'Connor, Orloff, Shaver 1999; Clement 1998) – which in this study will be dealt with in the context of financing long-term care through in-kind contributions. Here, positive autonomy requires that people are free to choose among different forms of contributing to the coverage of care needs. The choice is, for example, to decide freely among different options such as offering informal long-term care or participating in a regular employment relationship or combining the two options. For care receivers as well as informal care givers, autonomy requires that they are in a position to participate in the life of society in which they live. For care receivers there might be restrictions given by specific disabilities. Autonomy is then required to assure an adequate level of participation.

Positive autonomy requires choice sets and, hence, with regard to the provision of long-term care alternative settings, to provide care. This can be achieved either by offering a diversity of care opportunities or by offering money and by directing these benefits to those in need of care instead of directing it to agents or agencies. Offering cash might be favoured for arguments of personal freedom or negative autonomy, it might however conflict with the quality of care and the right to receive a certain amount of care. With regard to the principles used in the allocation procedure autonomy tends to be recognised by making need the only criterion, whereas other principles tend to have stigmatising or segregating effects.

In the finance of care positive autonomy requires equal choice sets with regard to contributions to the finance of long-term care. This becomes considerably important with regard to informal care-giving. Promoting personal autonomy would require a recognition of in-kind contributions made in the informal sector by, for example, establishing regular employment relationships, by recognising these contributions in a social protection system, or by offering social services enabling close family members to pursue a regular employment relationship outside the family.

The second major aspect of social integration are *social rights* and *responsibilities*. These are rights and responsibilities going beyond civil and political rights with the latter however being an integral prerequisite of social rights. Social rights might be enacted as legal rights (positive rights) or might be seen as ideal rights. For example, in a global perspective access to health care and education can be seen as such an ideal right. It is enacted as a legal right only in some countries, it might be accepted as an ideal right in many other countries even if actually not covered (see e.g. Plant 1998; Wilmot 1997).

With regard to long-term care the aspect of social rights is about the division of public and private responsibilities in the provision and the finance of long-term care as well as the quality of this division. Equal social rights and responsibilities would require that benefits are designed as rights instead of charity, that burdens are allocated recognising the various forms obligations might take (i.e. recognising the burden of informal unpaid care) and that individual dignity is preserved. Preserving individual dignity requires that resources are allocated without stigmatising or socially excluding effects on care receivers and their smaller social community. In long-term care such effects are more likely to occur in systems characterised by means-tested support for a minimum level, in systems differentiating support according to principles other than need-related principles or in systems offering substantial room for discretion.

Table 4.4 Equity objectives in welfare states

Equity objectives	Standard of reference – design of support
GUARANTEEING MINIMUM STANDARDS with regard to the availability of resources	minimum standard regarding availability of resources – support in case private means are not sufficient, social assistance principle
SUPPORTING LIVING STANDARDS after the occurrence of long-term care needs compared to the individual situation before that event	availability of resources before / after the occurrence of long-term care needs is compared – measures to reduce drops in the individual living standard related to the occurrence of long-term care needs, needs and living standard related
REDUCING HORIZONTAL INEQUALITIES in the availability of resources between those in need of long-term care and those not in need of long-term care	availability of resources between those in need of long-term care and those not in need of long-term care is compared (with regard to informal care-giving: between those providing and those not providing informal care) – measures to reduce inequalities between the two groups, support related to long-term care needs and informal long-term care provision
REDUCING VERTICAL INEQUALITIES between the economically better-off and the worse-off in society	availability of resources among the rich and the poor is compared – measures to reduce inequalities between the two groups by considering the economic status in providing resources and allocating burdens
ENHANCING PERSONAL AUTONOMY with regard to peoples' opportunities to freely choose among different options	opportunities to live an autonomous life – measures to enhance choice sets and to enhance financial and technical accessability regarding the different options
EQUALISING SOCIAL RIGHTS AND RESPONSIBILITIES	definition of private and public rights and responsibilities in long-term care – measures to clearly define and allocate rights and responsibilities in the provision and finance of long-term care

The level of information, of voluntariness and of competence might considerably constrain social integration (Wilmot 1997: 85). Information is a key prerequisite to translate autonomy and social rights from an objective as a declaration into real world practice. Choosing among different options requires information on the availability and the comparative quality of the various options. Voluntariness refers to freedom in making choices and to what extent it is a welfare state issue to enhance such choices, to maximise choices or to limit choices. Voluntariness is at the core of personal autonomy, that becomes a morally and ethically most demanding issue in the context of rationing care according to age or health status. Competence, finally, embodies two aspects. On the one hand, it requires to take measures to improve competence regarding choices and rights, on the other hand it points at the necessity to define competence and social integration with respect to health status in a given social and cultural environment.

In Table 4.4 equity objectives and the key indicators are summarised. The various objectives might be promoted by a wide range of methods. In translating equity objectives from theory or declaration into practice they may collide as well as harmonise with other societal objectives, such as freedom, efficiency, security and stability, peace or growth. And as Rae (1981: 5) puts it 'Perhaps indeed the idea against which equality must struggle most heroically is equality itself', pointing at the enormous variations in different equity objectives and the actual interpretations in real life decisions taking place on different societal levels. What is finally found in practice is the result of a number of issues discussed in the social choice and public choice literature, including issues such as ideology, attitudes and values, the role and power of parties and interest groups, etc.

4.3 Long-term care in Austria, Italy, the Netherlands and the United Kingdom: An overview

A brief overview to the long-term care systems in Austria, Italy, the Netherlands, and the United Kingdom will be given in this section in order to highlight the institutional mix and the policy mix in the respective countries. The following terminology will be used: 'residential care' (or 'institutional care') covering care in 'nursing homes' and 'residential homes'; 'domiciliary care' (or 'home care') covering 'home nursing' related to health aspects and 'home help' related to personal and domestic care; payments for care to care receivers and payments for care to informal care givers. (For more terminological details also see the Glossary.)

Long-term care in Europe: Some basic facts

Western European countries are characterised by similarities with regard to demographics and socio-demographic changes as well as with regard to the social and economic environment, which causes similar challenges to the welfare state design. (see Tables 4.5 and 4.6) As the prevalence of long-term care needs considerably increases with age, the number and the proportion of elderly people is an important indicator for present and future care-needs to be covered. In 1996 14.4 million people or 3.8% of the population in the European Union are 80 years of age or older. In the four

Table 4.5 Basic demographic data for Austria, Italy, the Netherlands and the United Kingdom

	A	I	NL	UK
Population by age group, 65+, total, 1995 (in 1000)	1,211.3	9,401.1	2,033.6	9,205.4
Population by age group, 80+, total, 1995 (in 1000)	312.3	2,292.3	475.8	2,334.7
65-79 as proportion of total population, 1996 (%)	11.4	12.7	10.2	11.7
80+ as proportion of total population, 1996 (%)	3.8	4.1	3.1	4.0
Forecast: Population by age group, 2010				
65-79 as proportion of total population (%)	12.8	14.7	11.2	11.7
80+ as proportion of total population (%)	4.7	5.8	3.8	4.3
Forecast: Population by age group, 2020				
65-79 as proportion of total population (%)	14.6	16.1	14.7	14.2
80+ as proportion of total population (%)	5.2	7.1	4.2	4.7
Increase in the population by age group, 1996-2010				
65-79 (%)	12	16	10	0
80+ (%)	24	41	23	8
Increase in the population by age group, 1996-2020				
65-79 (%)	28	27	44	21
80+ (%)	37	73	35	18

Source: Eurostat (1997); authors' calculations

countries covered by this study, the proportion of older people is above the average in Italy (4.1%) and in the United Kingdom (4.0%) and below average in the Netherlands (3.1%). In Austria the proportion of those 80 years and over lies with the European Union average. The same distribution can be found among those between 65 and 79 years of age. The European Union average is 11.7% with Italy above average, Austria and the

Netherlands below average and the United Kingdom at the same level as the European Union average.

Table 4.6 The social and economic environment in Austria, Italy, the Netherlands and the United Kingdom

	A	I	NL	UK
Gross domestic product (per capita $ 1998, current PPPs [1])	23,985	21,739	23,082	21,170
General government expenditure (% of GDP; 1996)	47.2	49.4	49.9	41.4
Social expenditure (% of GDP; 1996)	29.6	24.8	30.9	27.7
Female labour force participation [2]				
1988 (%)	53.7	43.2	50.6	63.7
1998 (%)	61.9	45.0	62.7	67.2
Part-time employment (% of total employment) [3]				
Women (1998)	22.8	22.4	54.8	41.2
Men (1998)	2.7	4.9	12.4	8.2
One-person households (as % of total households; 1990/91)	29.7	20.6	29.9	26.7
One-person households with householder aged 65+ (as % of all one-person households; figures from ECHP 1993)	46.4	55.2	38.0	53.9
Elderly people living alone (% of those aged 65+)	35 (1990)	31 (1990)	39 (1993)	38 (1991)

1) PPPs: Purchasing Power Parities are the rate of currency conversion which eliminates the differences in price levels between countries.
2) Female labour force of all ages divided by female population aged 15-64.
3) Part-time employment defined by a common definition of less than 30 usual-hours worked per week.

Source: OECD (1999); Ditch, Barnes, Bradshaw, Kilkey (1998); ÖSTAT 1999; OECD (2000)

Over the coming decades the proportion of elderly people in both these age-groups will increase in all of the countries studied here (see Table 4.5). In the year 2020 the number of those between 65 and 79 years of age will exceed the 14% share in all the countries, reaching 16.1% in Italy. The proportion of those 80 years and older will considerably increase until 2010 and again until 2020. In the year 2020 they will represent 4.2% of the population in the Netherlands, 4.7% in the United Kingdom, 5.2% in Austria and 7.1% in Italy. Compared to 1996 this represents an increase of between almost 20% (in the United Kingdom) and more than 70% (in Italy).

Given the fact that women are the main informal care givers (in particular with regard to informal care givers in their working age), and given the fact that in case of co-residence care the amount of informal care-giving is higher than in non-co-resident care, an increasing female labour force participation as well as an increase in solitary living will tend – other factors unchanged – to reduce the amount of informal care-giving. In the 1990s all the countries realised an increase of female labour force participation, which however was considerably lower in the United Kingdom (starting from a higher level) and in Italy which in 1997 showed the lowest level of female labour force participation in the European Union countries. On the other hand, women tend to be employed full-time in Italy and in Austria, whereas in the Netherlands and in the United Kingdom 55% and 40%, respectively, are part-time employed. Trends towards solitary living occur in all age-groups, with about one third of those aged 65 and over living on their own (see Table 4.6).

One has to deal with considerable problems of data availability and comparability when regarding the availability of long-term care services in the four countries (see chapter 4.1). However, an overview based on existing comparative as well as national data gives an indication regarding the 'ranking' of the four countries (see Table 4.7). Referring to other data sources (e.g. Jacobzone, Cambois, Chaplain, Robine 1999) provides quite different figures, however it does not change the 'ranking'. The number of beds in residential care settings compared to the number of elderly people is highest in the Netherlands followed by the United Kingdom, considerably lower in Austria, and lowest in Italy. These differences are not at all outweighed by differences in social service support. The distribution of social services in the four countries shows a very similar picture with highest support levels in the Netherlands followed by the United Kingdom. Figures for Austria and Italy have to be treated with caution, as there are considerable differences within these countries (which also is true to less extent for the United Kingdom). Both in Italy as well as in Austria the social service sector is growing, with some provinces or local areas with rather high service supply and other areas where these services are only in its infancy.

The picture, however, is quite different if one looks at payments for care. Such payments do play an important role in Austria and in Italy (where universal payment for care programmes exist), and in the United

Kingdom (with a mix of such programmes, some of them means-tested, offering payments to care receivers as well as care givers). In the Netherlands, payments for care only exist in the form of personal budgets which have been introduced on an experimental basis. Although still playing a minor role, they might become more important in the near future.

Table 4.7 Basic long-term care data

	A	I	NL	UK
Total spending on long-term care (1992-1995; % of GDP)	1.40	0.58	2.70	1.30
Public spending long-term care (1992-1995; % of GDP)	-	-	1.80	1.00
Public spending institutional care (1992-1995; % of public)	-	-	76	70
Private spending long-term care (1992-1995; % of total)	-	-	33	24
Residential care				
Residents as % of those 65+	4	2.5	9	5
Domiciliary care				
Home help recipients as % of those 65+	4 - 5	1	9 - 10	6 - 7
Payments for care	yes [1)]	yes [2)]	limited [3)]	yes [4)]

1) 'Pflegegeld'; benefits in cash to care receivers.
2) 'Indennità di Accompagnamento' and 'Assegno di Accompagnamento'; benefits in cash to care receivers.
3) Personal budgets; very limited number of recipients.
4) A variety of different programmes offering care money to care receivers as well as care givers.

Source: OECD (2000); OECD (1998); OECD (1996); Rostgaard, Fridberg (1998); Badelt, Leichsenring (2000); ISTAT (1997); Pesaresi, Simoncelli (1999)

Long-term care: The case of Austria

Long-term care in Austria has always been strongly based on family networks. Until 1993 the public support system in Austria was characterised by a decentralised structure of payments and institutional services, with provinces and communities being responsible for most of the long-term care matters. This resulted in considerable regional imbalances regarding residential and domiciliary care. In a number of provinces there were almost no social services available. In 1993 a payment for care programme initiated substantial changes in the system of care. Major policy objectives in Austria are the development of social services in the community, support for informal care, the assurance of high quality in care and cost containment.

The following discussion is based on references reviewing and evaluating the Austrian long-term care system, in particular Badelt, Leichsenring (2000), Barta, Ganner (1998), Badelt, Österle (2001b), Badelt, Holzmann-Jenkins, Matul, Österle (1997), Keigher (1997) as well as official publications (BMSG 2000; BMAGS 1999a; BMAGS 1999b). In addition, Austria has been covered by a number of comparative studies, including Leichsenring (1999), Weekers, Pijl (1998), Kalisch, Aman, Buchele (1998), Millar, Warman (1996), Wagner (1996), Evers, Leichsenring, Pruckner (1994). Benefit rates are given – if not otherwise stated – for the year 1999 in ATS and EURO following the EURO conversion rate: 1 EURO = 13.7603 ATS (Rates given in EURO do not represent official EURO benefit rates).

Residential care

As in the other countries, a major share of public money for long-term care has always been spent on care in residential care settings as well as in hospitals, offering care not only for severely disabled people but also for people who do not have access to alternative care settings due to supply shortage. Figures regarding the number of places in residential care settings vary between 41,000 and 65,000 (Badelt, Leichsenring 2000; Rubisch 1998). More than half of residential care settings are run by provincial or local public bodies, almost one third by non-profit organisations and the remaining by private for-profit institutions, which tend to be much smaller regarding the number of beds per unit (Badelt 1998). A lack of social services in the community as well as waiting lists in residential care settings resulted in a number of frail elderly people who are cared for in acute hospitals without need for acute care (Badelt, Holzmann, Matul, Österle 1996). More recently, however, considerable changes are taking place which lead to reduced waiting lists (Rudda 1998) and an increase in the proportion of more severely disabled people living in residential care settings. No significant changes are to be observed in the total number of beds (BMSG 2000).

Financing residential care settings is based on fees per day differentiating according to care needs. First of all, clients have to make out-of-pocket payments. Pensions as well as payments for care are directly transferred to these institutions (up to some pocket money). What is not covered through clients' contributions is covered by provinces or communities. These payments, following social assistance regulation in the provinces, may be recovered from clients' savings as well as from close family members. The respective regulations as well as the actual decisions vary considerably in the nine provinces (Barta, Ganner 1998). Overall, with the introduction of payments for care an important inter-governmental redistribution of burdens took place, lowering the proportion of costs in the residential care sector to be covered by social assistance. In 1997, about 50% could be recovered, whereas before the introduction of the payment for care programme the respective figure was about 25% (Pratscher, Stolitzka 1999).

Domiciliary care

Social services in the community still do not exist or are far from covering need for such services in a number of the nine provinces. In this respect the Austrian payment for care programme did not yet fundamentally change the existing system. But, according to a 'long-term care treaty' between the central government and the nine provinces the latter are obliged to develop a comprehensive community care system covering residential, semi-residential and domiciliary services until 2010 (BMAGS 1999b).

The provision of home nursing as well as home help services differs widely between provinces in terms of the level of provision as well as the organisation (Pratscher, Stolitzka 1999; BMAGS 1999b). Non-profit organisations are most important as providers of such services. Public bodies as well as for-profit organisations play a minor role in the actual provision. With the introduction of payments for care, competition has increased in some provinces, even if in many areas specific organisations still work in an almost monopolistic position. Regarding the co-ordination between various service providers, there is no nationwide concept, although a number of models evolved all over the country.

There is no systematic approach with regard to eligibility and access to these services, though some provinces use standardised forms for assessing needs. In the case of home nursing by qualified nurses, a referral from a physician is necessary in order to be reimbursed by the social health insurance fund. This reimbursement is based on a rather strict criteria covering only medical expenses such as administering injections or dressing wounds. Otherwise, home nursing as well as home help are funded by a combination of payments by provinces and municipalities (as a general subsidy or related to the number of clients) as well as by clients' co-payments (BMSG 2000). Co-payments became more widespread since payment for care programmes have been introduced. In general, co-payments are means-tested and increasingly related to the amount of the cash benefit. In one province, the provision of services is based on membership in the local home help organisation. Here, households have to pay membership fees instead of co-payments.

Payments for care (to care receivers)

In 1993 a payment for care programme ('Pflegegeld') was introduced for dependent people with at least 50 hours of care needs per month. Care needs are the only eligibility criterion. Payments which are directed to care receivers range from ATS 2,000 (EURO 145) per month in level one, to ATS 21,074 (EURO 1,532) per month in level seven. Level 1 is equivalent

Table 4.8 The Austrian payment for care programme

Depend. level	Attendance allowance (2001) ATS – EURO		Care needs (per month)	Recipients (Dec. 31, 1999)	
1	ATS 2,000	(EURO 145.3)	> 50 hours	53,547	*16.5%*
2	ATS 3,688	(EURO 268.0)	> 75 hours	126,326	*39.0%*
3	ATS 5,690	(EURO 413.5)	> 120 hours	58,329	*18.0%*
4	ATS 8,535	(EURO 620.3)	> 160 hours [1)]	46,227	*14.3%*
5	ATS 11,591	(EURO 842.4)	> 180 hours of intensive care	26,134	*8.1%*
6	ATS 15,806	(EURO 1,149.7)	> 180 hours of constant attendance	8,351	*2.6%*
7	ATS 21,074	(EURO 1,531.5)	> 180 hours of care, complete immobility	4,891	*1.5%*

1) Before 1999, level 4 required care needs exceeding 180 hours per month.

to care needs between 50 and 75 hours per month, level 7 is equivalent to care needs of more than 180 hours per month in combination with complete immobility (see Table 4.8). The evaluation of care needs is based on a medical certificate using standardised assessment procedure covering medical as well as household and personal needs. In dependency level 1 to

3 only the quantitative amount of care is taken into account, whereas evaluating dependency levels 4 to 7 also includes qualitative aspects. In general, the assessment is undertaken by medical staff of the authorities administering the payment for care programme. With the latest reform of the programme, care documentation has to be taken into account and informal care givers have to be consulted in the assessment procedure.

Payments for care are not means-tested and paid directly to care receivers. Beneficiaries are free to decide how to use the money. Only in case of 'improper use' can benefits in kind be offered as a substitute. In the case of residential care, the allowance is directly transferred – down to some pocket money – to the body in charge of the residential home. By the end of 1999, attendance allowances were paid to 323,805 disabled and frail elderly people, representing 4.0% of the Austrian population. About 45% are over the age of 80, 81% over the age of 60.

Payments for care (to informal care givers)

There are no direct payments of care to care givers. To some extent, however, payments made to care receivers are transferred to informal care givers. In general these payments cannot be seen as any form of income or compensation as they have to be used to cover extra expenses for care and in general do not even completely cover these extra expenses (Badelt, Holzmann-Jenkins, Matul, Österle 1997). In 1998 a possibility for coverage in the social pension insurance system at a lower rate for informal care givers was introduced. Those who care are eligible if they have given up regular employment in order to care for a close relative in need of care according to level 5 or higher (from 2001: level 4 or higher). In year 2000 just 271 people were covered under this scheme. Specific leave programmes for people offering informal long-term care do not exist. Just a one week leave for care is offered to anyone caring for a close relative. In the case of caring for children under the age of 12 another week of leave for care is available.

Informal care

Families and smaller social networks are playing a major role in long-term care. 90% of those receiving payments for care are cared for at home. Regarding the status quo of home nursing and home help services, this makes close family members the main care givers. In about 5% to 10% of all care arrangements, social services have to be seen as the main care giver. 80% of the main informal care givers are women, in particular daughters, daughters in law and partners. More than one third of the care givers are over the age of 60. 37% of those under the age of 60 are doing their care work alongside another formal job (Badelt, Holzmann-Jenkins, Matul, Österle 1997). A legal obligation of maintenance between close family members (spouses, children, parents) – with variations between the nine provinces – becomes particularly important in the case of financing care in residential care settings.

The finance of long-term care

Financing long-term care in Austria is based on taxes, social insurance contributions, out-of-pocket payments, private insurance contributions and informal care-giving without direct compensation. On the public level funding is primarily based on taxes. Social insurance contributions do play a very small role, as only medical home nursing is paid out of these funds and strict criteria are applied. The role of private insurance contributions in Austria is almost negligible, with the first private insurance solutions for long-term care occurring only in the 1990s.

Out-of-pocket payments play an important role in financing residential care and to less extent in financing social services. In the residential care sector personal income and payments for care of those cared for in residences – except for some pocket money – are directly transferred to these institutions. Additional costs covered by social assistance may be recovered from close family members. Different co-payment arrangements exist in the social service sector, differing across provinces and providers. They tend to be designed as a combination of income-related co-payments and a fixed amount per hour for those receiving payments for care (Leichsenring 1999). As has been shown above, long-term care very much remains on the shoulders of informal care givers. Potential indirect compensation from payments for care usually has to be used to cover extra costs of care and increasingly to pay for social services.

Long-term care: The case of Italy

Long-term care in Italy is strongly based on family and other informal care arrangements. The long-term care system is characterised by decentralised responsibilities and comparatively low numbers of people cared for by formal services. This, however, does not reflect the situation in the whole country, as there are enormous differences between regions and communities (Gori 2001). There are innovative forms of provision and in a number of cities in the north of the country formal service levels are as high as in the United Kingdom or even as in the Netherlands. A programme from 1992 ('Tutela della Salute degli Anziani') issued norms and guidelines for the development of long-term care. Although these are not legally binding for provinces and local administration, the programme can be seen as a national approach for a more systematic development of long-term care services. One of the important principles to be found in this document is the integration of health and social services.

Italy has long been neglected in international comparative work on long-term issues, but is increasingly recognised in recent years. The discussion below follows work by Gori (2001), Gori (2000), Mengani, Lamura, Melchiorre (1999), Beltrametti (1998), Longo (1997), ISTAT (1997) and Levorato, Rozzini, Trabucchi (1994). Work by Belletti, Keen (1999), Kalisch, Aman, Buchele (1998), Tester (1996), Hutten (1996a), Millar, Warman (1996), Facchini, Scortegagna (1993) and Glendinning, McLaughlin (1993) represent studies on the Italian long-term care system in a cross-country perspective. Benefit rates are given – if not otherwise stated – for the year 1999 in ITL and EURO following the EURO conversion rate: 1 EURO = 1,936.27 ITL. (Rates given in EURO do not represent official EURO benefit rates.)

Residential care

The situation regarding residential care in Italy is similar to other countries with respect to the broad variation in different existing types of residential care settings. The two main types are nursing homes ('Residenze Sanitarie Assistenziali') offering an extended range of health and social care, and residential homes ('Presidi Socio Assistenziali') with limited social care provision. It is a major policy concern to focus residential care on the more severely disabled elderly people and, hence, to bring residential care in line with the 'Residenze Sanitarie Assistenziali' type. About 2.7% of elderly people are cared for in residential care settings, representing a considerably lower proportion than in most other European countries. But there are substantial differences between the north and the south of the country. Whereas in many northern provinces more than 4% of those 65 years of age and older are cared for in residential care settings, the respective figure is below 1% in many southern provinces (Pesaresi, Simoncelli 1999). Slightly less then 50% of this population group are categorised as 'not self-sufficient'. The term 'self-sufficiency' is used if primary functions of daily living such as eating or walking are still independently done, but autonomous living is limited by other physical or mental restrictions or the unavailability of informal support (ISTAT 1997). Regarding the institutional mix, it is estimated that about 29% are public, 28% private but depending on public funding, whereas 43% are purely private homes (Belletti, Keen 1999).

There is a division between the health and the assistance aspect in the funding of these homes. Whereas health related care is financed by the regions, the assistance part has to be paid by clients. If clients do not have sufficient financial means and close relatives (children and other first-line relatives) are not capable to financially contribute, the local administration will finance the rest from social assistance funds.

Domiciliary care

There are no clear-cut responsibilities regarding domiciliary care in Italy, which is seen as one major causal factor for the fragmented and rather low service level. The main responsibility for social services is on the regional and local level, whereas the central government is only involved in funding projects in their experimental phase. Another vague dividing line is between the health sector organising domiciliary care within local health authorities ('Unità Sanitaria Locale') and the social service sector organising domiciliary care within local authorities. Service levels range between 7% of those 65 years of age and over receiving any kind of home nursing or home help in parts of the north of Italy, and below 1% in the south (Gori 2001).

In 1992 the concept of integrated home care ('Assistenza Domiciliare Integrata') was put forward, emphasising the integration of health related care and social services within the local health authorities. It requires collaboration between medical and nursing home care teams from the health sector and home help teams from the local authorities. This, of course, conflicted with already existing approaches organising home nursing and home help in the social service sector in the north of the country. A second approach which became important for the elderly, and in particular for terminally ill people, is the so-called home hospitalisation aimed at supporting people after hospitalisation and reducing the length of stay in hospitals. In November 2000 a national framework legislation on personal services passed the Parliament. The objective is to establish an integrated long-term care system, but criteria and procedures still have to be defined.

The assessment procedure does not require a formal referral and is usually undertaken by a geriatric evaluation committee (integrated home care), by a team from the hospital (hospitalisation at home) or social workers for home help services. As projects in their experimental phase, integrated home care as well as home hospitalisation were partly funded by national subsidies. Apart from this, domiciliary care is financed from global budgets of the communities (for social services) or from regions and local health authorities (for health related care). Budgets for health related expenditure are based on insurance contributions, general taxation as well as co-payments. Co-payment arrangements in the home help sector differ widely. Overall, it is estimated that 50% is paid by the clients themselves.

Payments for care (to care receivers)

There are two types of payments for care: the 'Indennità di Accompagnamento' (companion payment) and the 'Assegno di Accompagnamento' (companion cheque). The companion payment is a financial support for adult people with care needs, whereas the companion cheque is for disabled people under the age of 18. Potential beneficiaries have to apply to the local or provincial health units. Although the basic idea of the 'Indennita di Accompagnamento' was to support disabled people in the working age, it turned out to become a major form of support for elderly people. The payments are directed at the disabled or frail elderly person, who is free to use the money either to purchase formal services or to transfer money to informal care givers.

The maximum level of payments, which are not means-tested, is about ITL 800,000 (EURO 413) per month following national definitions of the degree of disability and care needs. The rate is set by the central government. Regions and provinces are, however, allowed to pay a higher rate. In 1997 the companion payment was paid to 860,000 people. Again, there are considerable variations between regions which can not be explained by variations in age structure and morbidity. The differences, relatively more and higher payments in the south of the country, are seen as an implicit response to the lack of services in this part of the country. (Gori 2001) More recently a number of regional and local authorities have – mostly on an experimental basis – introduced means-tested cash benefits explicitly designed as measures to support care in the family and to offer an alternative to public domiciliary services. (Morelli 1998) These payments are directed either to care receivers or informal care givers. Most of these new forms of cash options occurred in the north of the country.

Payments for care (to informal care givers)

There is no nationwide programme of direct payments to care givers. But care receivers are expected to use the cash benefit just described to either buy formal services or to pass it to informal care givers. Similar to Austria the payment, for care programme seems to be a national response to the pressing challenge of an increasing number of people in need of care without sufficient support from informal networks on the one hand and a lack of social services on the other hand. In some regions and local authorities cash payments are made to informal care givers offering additional financial support for families. Paid time-off from work for personal or family reasons is offered in some national collective agreements allowing short leaves of two or three days. In addition, some collective agreements offer extended unpaid leaves (up to four months) or part-time work. For those caring for a disabled child, 24 months leave are considered a contribution to the pension fund (Bettio, Prechal 1998).

Informal care

Informal care is playing a major role in long-term care in Italy. This is a consequence of a variety of factors, including the role of the family in the Italian society and the traditional model of extended family relations being still very important in the south of the country, the perception of care as a family obligation, and the low level of residential care and formal domiciliary care (Taccani 1999). As in Austria, there also is a legal obligation of maintenance between close family members. With regard to the distribution of care-giving burdens, evidence from Italy is in line with evidence from other countries. 78% of informal care givers are women, the majority daughters and daughters in law. On average, they spend 5.9 years on informal care-giving for frail elderly people (Lamura, et al. 1999).

The finance of long-term care

With regard to the division between public, private formal and private informal finance of long-term care, private solutions are more common in Italy than elsewhere. Informal care-giving plays the key role in the Italian long-term care system. Considerable out-of-pocket payments are required in residential as well as in domiciliary care. Finally, there is an important private sector covering care needs not met by public solutions, though the role of private insurance is negligible. Public finance is mainly based on tax revenues, and to a smaller extent on social insurance contributions.

Long-term care: The case of the Netherlands

Health and long-term care in the Netherlands is based on a two-tier health insurance system (combining social insurance and private insurance), and on a social health insurance scheme for the entire population. The latter scheme, the General Act on Exceptional Medical Expenses (AWBZ), also covers long-term care needs. This system was introduced in 1968. Whereas nursing homes were integrated from the beginning, homes for the elderly were integrated in the AWBZ system only in 1997 (with a transition period until 2001). The influence of central public bodies on long-term care issues is rather strong, including the general budgetary framework with spending limits, and the establishment of criteria for the allocation of services and quality standards. Long-term care provision is mainly in-kind oriented. Payments for care (personal budgets) introduced as an option to in-kind services do play a rather small role, although their introduction was generally regarded as successful. Cost-containment became an issue in the long-term care system earlier than in most other European countries. In addition, individual responsibility and choice, increased integration, flexibility and diversification of the system as well as the promotion of for-profit initiatives are major policy concerns.

Cross-country comparative work on the Netherlands, alongside the Scandinavian countries and the United Kingdom, is stronger than in Italy or Austria. The information used in this study mainly comes form comparative work, including work by Portrait, Lindeboom, Deeg (2000), Schuijt-Lucassen, Knipscheer (1999), Rostgaard, Fridberg (1998), Coolen, Weekers (1998), Weekers, Pijl (1998), Kalisch, Aman, Buchele (1998), Okma (1998), Tester (1996), Kerkstra (1996), Millar, Warman (1996) and Pijl (1993). Benefit rates are given in NLG and EURO following the EURO conversion rate: 1 EURO = 2.20371 NLG. (Rates given in EURO do not represent official EURO benefit rates.)

Residential care

The provision of residential care in the Netherlands is characterised by a decreasing number of people living in homes for the elderly and an increasing number of residents in nursing homes. Related to the number of those aged 65 and over, the proportion decreased for homes for the elderly and remained constant for nursing homes. Whereas the proportion of those living in homes for the elderly decreased from 8% to 5.5% (as a share of those 65 years of age and older) from 1981 till 1996, the number of those living in nursing homes remained almost unchanged (2.7%) (Rostgaard,

Fridberg 1998). This is because of cost containment policies aimed at reducing and targeting places in residential care settings by establishing a 7% rule (limiting the number of beds to 7% of the elderly population in the region) and the introduction of user fees in nursing homes. In general, differences between the two types of residences diminish, while alternative forms of residential and semi-residential care occur. Most of the residential care settings are run by non-profit organisations, to a very small extent by public bodies and an almost negligible extent by for-profit organisations.

Financing residential care is mainly based on AWBZ funds. This is the case for nursing homes, although user fees related to income have been introduced. Homes for the elderly are in a transition period. Up to now residents had to pay fees out of their income combining a fixed and a means-tested fee. In addition, private savings had to be used, without a family obligation to do so. The difference was paid by local authorities out of social assistance funds. For the future financing regulations in residential care are being harmonised under AWBZ, that is coverage by public funds plus means-tested co-payments.

Domiciliary care

Social services caring for the clients in their own home (home nursing and home help services) are organised within regional organisations, which became more integrated home care organisations recently. Most of the services are run by non-profit organisations in an almost monopolistic position on a regional level. The importance of private for-profit home care organisations is not substantial, though recently they were explicitly supported by reserving part of the budget for such organisations. Competition therefore might become more important, also because there are waiting lists in the home help sector and people having personal budgets at their disposal (see below).

Access to services is universal with no formal referral required. The assessment of care needs is undertaken by special assessment teams covering home nursing, home help as well as care in residential settings. Despite universal access there is no individual right to receive home help services (which exists for home nursing). Strict budget control by the government, therefore, led to restrictions and waiting lists in the home help sector. The proportion of those 65 years of age or older receiving domiciliary care increased from 7.7% in 1983 to almost 10% in 1996 (Rostgaard, Fridberg 1998). Home nursing as well as home help services are mainly paid out of AWBZ budgets transferring money to Home Care Organisations which in turn pay providers. To a smaller extent means-tested co-payments and membership fees have to be made, counting for about 10% of total expenditure.

Payments for care (to care receivers)

After an experimental phase, personal budgets were introduced in 1995 as an alternative to in-kind services for those people to be expected in need of care for an extended period of more than 3 months. Those interested have to contact the regional office of the medical care insurance. There is no formal referral required, the assessment is the same as with in-kind benefits, and takes into account to what extent family members are able to support the person in need of care. The Social Insurance Bank takes care of the administrative tasks like informing and advising budget-holders and paying salaries to helpers employed by personal budgetholders. Although personal budgets have been evaluated as a rather successful approach in redesigning long-term care policies (see Coolen, Weekers 1998; Weekers, Pijl 1998), the overall spending limit for personal budgets is still rather small compared to the whole budget for home care (about 3-5%).

Personal budgets are funded by AWBZ funds transferred to local Home Care Organisations. The maximum amount a client can get is based on the assessment of hours of care needs and the tariffs for the different kinds of services. In December 2000 the respective tariffs range between NLG 20.70 (EURO 9.40) per hour for domestic help and NLG 96.60 (EURO 43.80) for specialised nursing. From the personal budget a means-tested co-payment is deducted. In the year 2000 the programme covered about 13,000 people in need of care. Just a small amount of NLG 2,400 NLG (EURO 1,089) per year is at the disposal of the person in need of care for out-of-pocket expenses. The major part is used for paying home help and personal care services from for-profit and non-profit providers and the so-called alpha-helpers employed by care receivers (Coolen, Weekers 1998).

Payments for care (to informal care givers)

There are no payments of care to care givers and the amount of money from personal budgets that is at the disposal of the person in need of care is comparatively small, hence limiting the possibilities to transfer money to informal carers. There is no statutory scheme in the Netherlands that gives someone the opportunity of leave for care. But there are arrangements in a number of agreements between social partners regarding leaves for care for a sick relative or so-called emergency leaves. These time off work arrangements are partly paid, partly unpaid. A further opportunity is offered by the so-called career leave (2 – 6 months), which might be used for care. However, the level of benefits – paid out of the unemployment fund – is rather small and below the assistance level (Bettio, Prechal 1998).

Informal care

Maintenance in case of long-term care needs between close family members is not established as a legal obligation in the Netherlands as it is the case in Italy or in Austria. Still, informal care plays an important role in domestic care and to some extent in personal care, although the extent to which care is offered in the formal sector is considerably higher than in the other three countries. But there is an increase in 'implicit' obligations of family members because of spending limits in public support and the objective to support people in their own home. Limitations in access to residential care and the existence of waiting lists in home help services are a clear indication of this trend. There have, however, also been support programmes including the introduction of short-term stays in institutional settings, the introduction of career breaks, information centres for carers and support by professional carers.

The finance of long-term care

Long-term care in the Netherlands is mainly covered by AWBZ. Only homes for the elderly have been financed mainly out-of-pocket and from state subsidies. But these care settings will be fully integrated in AWBZ in the near future. Funding of AWBZ is based on tax-related contributions as well as subsidies from the state. The overall budgets include fixed spending limits determined annually by the central government. With the integration of the different types of residential care settings in AWBZ the role of out-of-pocket payments will be limited in all sectors to means-tested co-payments. But, the amount of these co-payments has increased in recent years. The role of private insurance solutions is negligible as in all other European countries. Informal care-giving without compensation plays an important role. Consequently, a considerable burden remains to informal care givers. It is estimated that informal care in the Netherlands is about eight times the amount of formal home help hours (Kwekkeboom cit. in Rostgaard, Fridberg 1998).

Long-term care: The case of the United Kingdom

Long-term care in the United Kingdom is separate from health care with strong local responsibilities in long-term care. Developments in the 1980s and those following the 1989 White Paper 'Caring for People' and the NHS and Community Care Act 1990 shifted major long-term care responsibilities to local authorities. This shift is characterised by emphasising domiciliary care services, by increasingly discretionary service domains and independent service providers in the private sector (Glendinning 1998b). The development of care management and assessment procedures was aimed at optimising appropriate care packages under increasing financial and organisational constraints (Mannion, Smith 1998). Various long-term care related cash benefits in the United Kingdom follow different eligibility criteria and are directed either to those in need of care or to informal care givers. Major recent policy concerns, also addressed by The Royal Commission on Long Term Care (1999), include the finance of care, the support of care in the community, a further shift from public to private (non-profit and for-profit) provision, an integration of services, and the recognition of the role of informal carers.

The following discussion of the long-term care system in the United Kingdom is based on Bond, Buck (1999), Glendinning (1998b), Rostgaard, Fridberg (1998), Weekers, Pijl (1998), Kalisch, Aman, Buchele (1998), Rowlands (1998), Glendinning, Schunk, McLaughlin (1997), Tester (1996), Richards (1996), Millar, Warman (1996), Hutten (1996b), Leat, Ungerson (1994), Lewis (1994), Baldock (1993); Glendinning, McLaughlin (1993) as well as research undertaken in the context of The Royal Commission on Long Term Care (1999). Benefit rates (as effective from April 2000) and other monetary information is given in GBP and EURO following an average exchange rate (average 2000) of: 1 EURO = 0.61 GBP.

Residential care

Residential care in the United Kingdom is run by public as well as private organisations. Since the 1980s the role of public providers declined, whereas the role of for-profit providers increased and non-profit providers held their position. In 1996 almost 64% of residents are living in private homes, whereas just 21% and 15%, respectively, are living in homes provided by local authorities and the voluntary sector (Rostgaard, Fridberg 1998). The process of contracting-out residential care was supported by economic incentives and the requirement to spend a certain amount in the independent sector. After an increase in the number of people living in residential care settings until the beginning of the 1990s, numbers slightly fell. In general, residents nowadays are older and have extended care needs. The assessment for access to residential care is combined with the general assessment of care needs by multi-disciplinary assessment teams.

The regulation of the finance of care has been changed in 1993. Those whose capital assets exceed GBP 16,000 (EURO 26,230) as well as those with sufficient regular income have to pay the fees in full. Otherwise people have to make a financial contribution. Means-testing takes income, assets as well as Income Support or other social security benefits into account. Only capital assets below GBP 10,000 (EURO 16,393) are ignored. There is no legal obligation for relatives to pay, but there is a principle of liability between spouses. They may be asked to contribute to costs, can however not be forced to do so. On average, one third of costs is covered by clients' payments (The Royal Commission on Long Term Care 1999).

Domiciliary care

Home nursing is part of the National Health Service and accordingly organised. Home help services are organised by local authorities acting as purchasers and – though decreasingly – as providers, voluntary organisations as well as private for-profit organisations. Following the objective of splitting the role of purchasing and provision, the role of private for-profit as well as non-profit organisations became more important. But local authorities are still the main providers of domiciliary care services in the United Kingdom.

The assessment is increasingly based on standardised assessment forms and undertaken by a social worker of the local authorities, a home care team, or a care manager. In the decision over care arrangements, the possibility to stay in the home as well as clients' and carers' preferences have to be considered. The availability of sufficient financial means can be taken into account, denying public services for the more wealthy clients. In 1996, almost 6% of those 65 years of age and older and 17% of those 85 years of age and older received home help (Rostgaard, Fridberg 1998). Whereas the number of people receiving home help decreased considerably in the 1990s, the number of hours per client increased. This reveals a concentration on personal care (and less on domestic care) and on those people with higher care needs, indicating a similar development as observed in the Netherlands.

Nursing care is fully covered by central government money. Home help is financed out of local funds (based on grants from the central government and local taxes). Whether services are paid out of these funds depends on needs assessment and means-testing, which varies considerably between local areas. There is a shift towards co-payment regulations and towards means-tested fees instead of flat rate payments. It is estimated that co-payments count for about 10% of total costs (Rostgaard, Fridberg 1998).

Payments for care (to care receivers)

The payment for care system in the United Kingdom is characterised by a variety of such programmes, differing in objectives and target groups. The Attendance Allowance is a tax-free and not means-tested social security benefit for people who are 65 and over in need of personal care. The intention of the allowance is to cover extra expenses related to these needs. Claimants must have been in need of help for at least six months. For the terminally ill there are special regulations. The Attendance Allowance – as effective from April 2000 – is either GBP 35.80 (EURO 58.70) per week or GBP 53.55 (EURO 87.80) per week for people needing help by day and by night. In 1997, 14,5% of those over the age of 65 years received this benefit.

The Disability Living Allowance was introduced in 1992 for people under the age of 65 (replacing the former attendance allowance for this age group). Claimants must have needed personal care for three months and must be expected to need such care for at least six more months. The Disability Living Allowance, which is not means-tested, consists of two components: The care component which is between GBP 14.20 and GBP 53.55 (EURO 23.30 – 87.80) per week and the mobility component which is between GBP 14.20 and GBP 37.40 (EURO 23.30 – 61.30) per week. In 1997 there were 1.768,000 recipients.

The so-called Constant Attendance Allowance is paid for those whose disablement pension is payable at the 100% rate. This allowance is not income-related. The condition for receiving Constant Attendance Allowance is the receiver's disability requiring daily care and attendance. According to care needs, the normal maximum rate is GBP 43.80 (EURO 71.80). In addition, there is a lower part-time rate GBP 21.90 (EURO 35.90) and two higher rates at GBP 65.70 (EURO 107.70) and GBP 87.60 (EURO 143.60) for exceptionally severe disablement.

Benefits from the Independent Living Fund 1993 are restricted to people in the ages between 16 and 65 living alone or with another person unable to provide care. Allowances are based on an assessment of care needs, but very much restricted in a number of additional respects. Claimants may only have a very small amount of private savings and an income that is too small to cover care needs not covered by other benefits. The benefit has to be used to employ one or more people (not close relatives living in the same household) for support in personal or domestic care. The fund works in partnership with local authorities. The number of beneficiaries is rather small, but they tend to have very high care needs. On average beneficiaries receive GBP 185 (EURO 303.30) per week, the maximum rate is GBP 300 (EURO 491.80).

Income support is for those whose income from whatever source is below a minimum level set by the Parliament. Before 1993 Income Support was a main source for paying fees for residence in private homes. Today there is only the standard rate available (except for those who have been living in private homes before 1993). There are, however, a number of specific premiums recognising extra needs among receivers of Income Support. These premiums include the Disabled Child Premium, the Disability Premium, the Severe Disability Premium and the Carer Premium (for the latter see below).

The Severe Disablement Allowance is made to working age people (16 – 65 years of age) who have not been able to work for at least 28 weeks because of an illness or disability, but do not have access to sickness or invalidity benefits. The assessment is made by a general practitioner. From April 2000 the benefit is GBP 40.80 (EURO 66.90) per week plus an extra benefit between GBP 4.50 and GBP 14.20 (EURO 7.40 – 23.30) per week depending on age and an extra benefit for dependent people living in the same household. The Severe Disability Premium (GBP 40.20 / EURO 65.90) is a means-tested benefit for people with a high level of care needs living alone or with a person that does not receive the Invalid Care Allowance (see below).

Direct Payments were introduced in 1997 offering local authorities the opportunity to make direct payments to people in need of care instead of in-kind services. The programme is directed at those between 18 and 65, and at those over 65 if they entered the programme under this age. Whether such a programme is established and to what extent such payments are made is regulated on the local level.

Payments for care (to informal care givers)

The Invalid Care Allowance is paid to informal care givers in the working age (16 – 65 years), but not to those in full-time education. The person cared for must receive an Attendance Allowance or a Disability Living

Allowance at a middle or higher rate. Caring has to exceed 35 hours per week. The idea of the programme is to replace lost earnings. The Invalid Care Allowance is not means-tested, but taxable. The basic rate is GBP 40.40 (EURO 66.20) per week from April 2000, but individual circumstances such as other dependent persons living in the same household are taken into account.

The Carer Premium is a means-tested allowance for informal carers in receipt of Income Support. From April 2000 the Carer Premium rate is GBP 14.15 (EURO 23.20) per week. With the Home Responsibilities Protection the right to Basic Retirement Pension is protected if carers are engaged in caring for at least 35 hours a week for a person receiving benefits because of sickness or disability. Cash benefits tend to be used to cover care-related costs rather than as a compensation for informal care (Glendinning 1992) which corresponds with results from the evaluation of the Austrian payment for care programme (Badelt, Holzmann-Jenkins, Matul, Österle 1997).

Informal care

The fiscal value of informal care was recently estimated to be at least as 5 times as high as total public spending (Glendinning, Schunk, McLaughlin 1997). In contrast to most other European countries a number of studies show a higher proportion of male care givers. According to Rowlands (1998) 61% of carers (devoting more than 20 hours per week to caring) are women and 39% men, caring mainly for spouses or parents. 73% of informal carers are under the age of 65 and hence – potentially – have to combine informal care-giving and formal employment. Other than in Austria and in Italy, there is no family obligation in the United Kingdom to care for an older relative. However, recent developments in residential and domiciliary care regulations allow local authorities to consider the availability of informal care in the assessment of care needs and the decision over the care arrangement. This tends to increase family responsibilities either for informal care-giving or for the arrangement of formal private solutions. On the other hand, there also is an increased awareness of the precarious situation of many informal carers which has been recognised more than in other countries through the 1996 Carers Act and the Carers National Association, which is engaged in advising and supporting informal carers as well as in lobbying.

The finance of long-term care

In general, public finance of long-term care is tax-based. Residential and domiciliary care are mainly funded by central government money transferred to local authorities as grants. There is not one single grant but a combination of grants related to different variables such as demographic factors or the support of specific services. Local authorities may supplement these funds by their own taxes, but are restricted in this respect. Whereas public finance of in-kind services is fully tax-based there are contributory systems for some cash benefits, combining contributions from employers and employees.

Out-of-pocket payments play an increasing role. Apart from nursing care, clients are now charged for all in-kind services. Parallel to shifting responsibilities to local authorities there are considerable local differences, despite the fact that the authorities have to follow guidelines specifying arrangements for user fees, for example that there should be no user fees for people on cash assistance benefits. Overall, user fees account for about 20% of total expenditure in residential and domiciliary care, whereas the proportion is considerably higher in residential care.

The increase of private providers in long-term care, in particular in the residential care sector, is substantial. Private long-term care insurance is playing an increasing role in the debate how to finance long-term care in the future. Presently, it plays a minor role in the actual long-term care system in the United Kingdom as in all other European countries. But also its potential in designing future long-term care finance is regarded as limited (see e.g. The Royal Commission on Long Term Care 1999). Although there is no legal obligation of maintenance for dependent family members, an enormous amount of care-giving is undertaken in the informal sector. Reforms in the 1990s have partially even shifted responsibilities back from the public sector to the private sphere.

5 Equity Choices in Long-Term Care: A Comparative Perspective

Part 5 aims at comparatively analysing similarities and differences in equity choices in the long-term care systems in Austria, Italy, the Netherlands and the United Kingdom and to contrast these choices with equity objectives in the welfare state. In chapters 5.1 and 5.2, equity choices are compared with respect to resources and burdens to be shared, among whom the resources and burdens are allocated and according to which principles allocation takes place. Whereas in chapter 5.1 the focus is on equity choices in the provision of care, chapter 5.2 focuses on equity choices in the finance of long-term care. In chapter 5.3 the results for the two spheres are brought together in the light of basic equity objectives of the welfare state.

5.1 Equity choices in the provision of long-term care

All the countries covered by this study are characterised by a division of responsibilities between public bodies on the various levels. The role of public bodies on the regional and local level in the provision and in the regulation of provision is rather strong compared with other social policy fields. Whereas central public bodies are in charge of cash benefits, regulations regarding financing long-term care and basic regulations regarding the provision of care, regional and local public bodies are in charge of provision and/or regulation of residential care settings and social services. The role of informal care-giving has long been almost ignored in all the countries but is nevertheless the main source of care-giving. Only in recent years is there more awareness of informal long-term care which – to some extent – is also reflected in policy initiatives, such as the introduction of payment for care programmes, the recognition of informal care-giving in social protection schemes, or the establishment of carers associations.

The following discussion investigates equity choices in long-term care policies in Austria, Italy, the Netherlands, and the United Kingdom focusing on the provision of care. The analysis will follow the framework developed in part 3 of the study (see Table 3.2), that is by analysing the three basic elements of equity choices: what is to be shared, among whom, and according to which principles. Equity choices as designed or as influenced by the public sector will be studied. Choices within or by other sectors such as families will not be analysed per se, but examined in the way they are affected by public equity choices. This approach will highlight and clarify how basic welfare state ideas about long-term care are translated into long-term care practice. In chapter 5.3 these choices, together with equity choices made in the finance of long-term care, will be contrasted with equity objectives identified in chapter 4.2.

What resources?

Welfare state approaches in long-term care in terms of resources include, broadly speaking, benefits in-kind and cash benefits as well as regulation. Part 4 has given an overview regarding long-term care resources provided in Austria, Italy, the Netherlands and the United Kingdom. According to the division of private and public responsibilities, public support for in-kind provision is strongest in the Netherlands and lowest in Italy. Payments for care, however, provide an almost opposite picture. Cash payments are highest in Austria. They also play an important role in Italy and in the United Kingdom, whereas cash benefits are of limited importance in the Netherlands (see Table 4.7).

These resources are intermediate means to achieve final objectives. The 'final goods' public policies might be aimed at are the *final outcome*, the *use* of specific services in the formal or informal sector, *access* to care, as well as *choice* between various care arrangements (see part 3).

Quite clear distinctions can be figured out in the four countries regarding the *use* of specific services. Whereas in Italy and Austria there is a legal obligation for family members to care between adults, this does not exist in the United Kingdom and in the Netherlands (Millar, Warman 1996). In Austria this obligation covers spouses, parents and children, in Italy other first-line relatives too. In both countries regulations do not refer to the actual provision of care, but the 'obligation of maintenance'. Financial sources from relatives may be used to recover public expenditure for publicly provided services. In practice, there is considerable room for discretionary decision in both countries. Although there is no explicit legal obligation of family members in long-term care in the United Kingdom, there is an increasing recognition of the informal care potential in the assessment of care needs and in the decision over the care arrangement.

With regard to the use of residential versus domiciliary care settings there is a strong trend towards care at home in all the countries, favoured for arguments of cost containment and social integration. This, however, addresses not just the question of residential vs. domiciliary care, but broader issues about the optimal care setting between care in hospitals and care at home and about co-ordination and co-operation between different settings (see e.g. Schulz-Nieswandt 1999; Tester 1996). The reduction of hospital days is a major cost containment concern in health policies all over Europe including attempts to seek appropriate and more cost-effective ways of supporting long-term care needs. In this respect, most European countries have been successful in reducing hospital days, whereas the response on the side of residential or domiciliary care settings was more limited (Tester 1996; Glendinning 1998b; Coolen, Weekers 1998).

In the residential care sector a concentration on those with more severe care needs can be observed in all the countries, and even a reduction of the number of beds in the Netherlands and to a smaller extent in the United Kingdom (Rostgaard, Fridberg 1998). Historically, home nursing and home help became more widespread in the Netherlands and in the United Kingdom before this was the case in Austria and in Italy. In Austria – apart from some of the provinces – residential care has been seen as the major public response to the long-term care issue until the beginning of the 1990s. Italy is characterised by low supply levels in the residential as well as in the domiciliary care sector, although there are considerable differences within the country (see chapter 4.3). At the same time, even in Italy it is estimated that 20% of those living in nursing homes could be cared for appropriately at home (Montanelli 1998).

Payment for care programmes are a trend to be observed in long-term care policies in a number of European countries. The impact on the care arrangement depends on the actual design of such programmes as well as the overall long-term care system. Payment for care programmes without restrictions regarding use of these benefits – as it is the case in Austria, in Italy, and partly in the United Kingdom – emphasise 'choice'. Other payment for care programmes restrict 'choice' to buy services in the formal sector or a segment of the formal sector, as it is the case in the Netherlands. Hence, payment for care programmes reflect different public objectives and choices, either directed at the use of specific services (freedom of choice is restricted to providers within this service sector), or directed at offering choice between different kinds of services (including the formal and the informal sphere). However, whether such choice really exists in practice also depends on the development of services in the formal sector as well as the extent to which payments for care are available. In all the countries, payments for care have to be seen only as a financial contribution to cover long-term care expenditure. This is even true when benefits are relatively high, as in Austria where these benefits are explicitly defined as a contribution to cover extra expenses of care (see e.g. Badelt, Holzmann-Jenkins, Matul, Österle 1997; Glendinning 1992). In the Netherlands cash benefits for care play a minor role. Here, choice is based on a broader set of in-kind services. Among the countries studied here, the number of people provided with services from the residential and the domiciliary care sector is highest in the Netherlands.

Access describes the opportunity to use, but not the actual use of services. The levels of provision in Italy and in Austria are considerably lower than in the Netherlands and in the United Kingdom. In fact, access to domiciliary care still does not even exist in many parts of Italy (e.g. Gori 2001) or is limited in parts of Austria (BMAGS 1999b). Using differences in waiting lists as an indicator of unmet need – that is interpreting waiting lists as an indicator of the opportunity to use such services – is misleading, as a number of studies have shown that demand in long-term care is greatly determined by the supply level in specific sectors (e.g. Kemper 1992).

Payments for care can be seen as an intermediate means to enable access to the actual provision of care. A number of payment for care programmes evolved in the 1990s, among the countries studied here, most prominently in Austria where the programme offers comparatively higher payments to a larger number of people. Potential and risk of such payments are discussed rather controversially (e.g. Tilly 1999; Glendinning, Schunk, McLaughlin 1997; Ungerson 1995; Evers, Pijl, Ungerson 1994; Ungerson 1993). Finally, the implications will depend on the details in the design of payments for care as well as the overall design of a long-term care system, and hence the mix of resources and principles used to allocate these resources. Cash benefits increase purchasing power in the hands of potential clients (or informal carers) and will tend to create more demand for services either within or from outside the narrow informal care network. However, as payments are just a contribution to cover extra-costs of care, they first tend to be used to cover these extra-costs and to increase demand for services either in the wider informal sector, in a low paid formal sector or in a subsidised formal sector. This can either create an incentive to withdraw or to reduce formal employment (because of additional financial resources available). It may, however, also make it possible to combine working in the formal labour market and informal caring (by paying for social services). In addition, payments for care may have important effects on aspects of independent living and autonomy, and hence the idea of social integration.

Outcome, the final objective in long-term care, is rather difficult to approach. Care is about nursing, as well as assistance and support in health-related matters, in personal and domestic activities. And care is about the actual task as well as the emotional relationship. The contribution of long-term care policies to the final outcome is to be found in the quantity and quality of care. This includes a wide range of variables, such as the response of care arrangements to individual preferences, the qualification of care givers or the opportunity of independent living under the constraints of limiting conditions in health.

Long-term care policies tend to approach the broader issue of the final outcome in at least two ways: quality standards and a range of service alternatives. Standardised needs assessment and standards for the actual service provision in the formal sector (such as professional qualifications, guidelines and care plans, the number of beds in residential care settings or the number of qualified home nurses related to the elderly population) are seen as major approaches to support the final outcome. The fact that this policy concern evolves at the same time as cost containment concerns suggests that such measures are aimed at securing certain standards of quality under more rigid economic constraints. At the same time they might have an equalising effect across institutions and local areas, at least for some basic standards. Though on very different levels, in all the countries a broadening of service alternatives (e.g. semi-residential settings) can be observed at the same time as increasing restrictions regarding access to specific forms of provision (Pacolet, Bouten, Lanoye, Versieck 1999a).

Among whom?

Following the overall objective of guaranteeing a specific quantity and quality of care, public policies in the provision of care may be directed at *individuals* as the final target group as well as *individuals*, *local areas* or *institutions* as intermediate target groups. *Local units* have traditionally been strong in Italy and in Austria, where in-kind benefits are a regional or local responsibility. In Austria, by means of a treaty between the state and the provinces on the development of social services, local variations shall be reduced until 2010 (BMAGS 1999b; Barta, Ganner 1999). In Italy, except for nation-wide cash benefits and an increasing debate on the issue, local variations are still enormous (e.g. Gori 2001). In the United Kingdom, reforms in the 1980s and the 1990s have shifted responsibilities to local authorities and increased variations in service provision between local areas (Glendinning 1998b; Walker 1995).

Regional and local areas, or segments in the private institutional mix, are becoming the focal unit if central government money is specifically transferred to these segments, as it is the case in the United Kingdom and in the Netherlands. Consequences in terms of supply levels in these two countries are rather different, caused by differences in additional policy measures to guarantee specific standards across the country. Whereas in the United Kingdom an increase in territorial inequalities is observed, this is not the case in the Netherlands (Glendinning 1998b; Coolen, Weekers 1998).

Specific *institutions* or specific segments in the institutional mix might be preferably subsidised in order to shift expenditure levels between the residential and the domiciliary care sector or between the public and the private formal sector. Examples are the 7% rule in the Netherlands (beds in residential care settings are only subsidised up to 7 beds per 100 elderly people in a specific region over the age of 65), spending limits in the Netherlands, or the reservation of public funds for the independent sector in the United Kingdom.

The role of *family members* as carers in the four countries has been briefly described above and will be touched upon again in discussing the finance of long-term care (see chapter 5.2). Apart from rather clear differences in the 'obligation' to care, an increasing recognition of the role of informal carers – in terms of addressing informal care-giving in the debates – can be observed in all the countries. But actual support for informal care-giving with regard to long-term care is still low compared to care-giving for children (Bettio, Prechal 1998). Some first steps have been taken more recently to approach individuals in their role as informal long-term carers. In general, these approaches have to be seen as cost-containment measures and as a means to strengthen the role of informal care-giving in potential care arrangements. This becomes increasingly important with shifting the policy focus from residential care to domiciliary care. The socio-economic situation of informal carers is recognised to a much smaller extent in these efforts, if at all. In all the countries except the Netherlands payment for care programmes are seen – among other objectives – as direct or indirect financial support and an incentive for informal care-giving. As evidence shows, the incentive arises not from payments regarded as financial compensation for the work done in the informal sector, but from regarding payments as recognition of informal care work enabling extra-costs of care to be covered (Glendinning 1998b; Badelt, Holzmann-Jenkins, Matul, Österle 1997). Care leave programmes are an additional approach to promote informal care-giving, although the importance of existing short-term leave programmes is limited in the case of long-term care. Extended leave programmes in the Netherlands and partly in Italy are not designed as social rights, but restricted to collective agreements.

How?

To what extent shares of specific resources are allocated is determined by a wide range of principles of allocation. These principles not only determine whether someone receives a share of the resources or not, but also the amount of resources allocated. The basic principles according to which resources in long-term care may be shared are need, time-related, status, economic, mixed and implicit principles.

Need seems to be the most adequate allocation principle with respect to equity considerations in the provision of health and social care. And in fact, need is probably the most widespread principle of allocating resources in long-term care. On the other hand, need is far from being a clear-cut single principle. Need principles are based on morbidity or disability measures, the inability to carry out certain activities of daily living, the amount of time needed to support people or the ability to benefit from support. In addition, needs measurement differs according to those who are involved in the assessment procedure.

Principles of need can be found for all forms of provision in all the countries looked at in this study. In the Netherlands needs assessment for all different forms of provision – residential care, domiciliary care, and personal budgets – is undertaken by the same assessment team, which also decides the care arrangement. To some extent this is also true for Italy and the in-kind sector in the United Kingdom. In Austria those responsible for the assessment are general practitioners (in case of payments for care as well as home nursing to be financed by social insurance funds), in the case of residential or domiciliary care this is a nurse or an assessment team from the respective institution. If someone is applying for a place in a residential care setting, some of these institutions are increasingly assessing whether domiciliary care would be adequate and possible, but there is no such general approach in Austria.

In Italy and to less extent in Austria, coverage with residential and domiciliary care only exists in part of the country or is rather limited. Apart from these restrictions, assessment procedures and the decision whether a person receives home care or a place in a residential care setting, depends on policies on the regional and local level as well as on the approach by the respective providers. Payment for care programmes in both countries are based on national definitions of disability or care needs. Evidence supports the conclusion that a high take-up rate and a high level of equal payments according to need is achieved in Austria, even more so as there have recently been further adaptations and clarifications in the definition of needs (BMAGS 1999a). In Italy considerable variations between different areas occur, which cannot be related to differences in morbidity and disability (Gori 2001).

Table 5.1 Need-related principles in allocating resources

	Austria	Italy	Netherlands	United Kingdom
Allocating places in nursing homes and allocating social services	no standardised approach; definitions vary between provinces and providers; increasingly referring to needs assessment in the payments for care scheme	no standardised approach; definitions vary between provinces and providers; some trends towards needs assessment by one team to decide upon various forms of in-kind benefits	needs assessment by one assessment team for the whole range of benefits; national standards preventing territorial inequalities but causing some inflexibility; increasingly used to decide not just on the extent of specific support, but on the optimal care package	towards needs assessment by one assessment team; increasingly used to decide on the optimal care package; shifting responsibilities to local managers causes local variations
Allocating cash benefits	standardised needs-assessment (national standards) as the only criterion of eligibility; non-need-related variations are small	standardised needs-assessment (national standards) as the only criterion of eligibility; local variations in take-up-ratios		needs-assessment varies according to benefit; additional principles of allocation

In the Netherlands and in the United Kingdom needs assessment is increasingly used not just to decide upon the extent of specific support, but to decide on the optimal care package, including the decision of residential vs. domiciliary care. In the 1990s, responsibilities in the United Kingdom have been increasingly shifted to care managers. Actual and potential consequences of local responsibilities under considerable financial constraints are heavily debated with regard to efficiency and equity concerns, in particular territorial inequalities (see e.g. Ellis, Davis, Rummery 1999; Leat, Perkins 1998; Baldock 1997; Davies 1987). In the Netherlands, stricter national regulation prevented such geographical variations. On the other hand, this is seen as a major cause for inflexibility in the long-term care system in the Netherlands, addressed more recently by emphasising provider networks (Coolen, Weekers 1998).

Although the definition of need is central to designing and analysing social policies, there is a significant lack of information on how different assessment procedures do influence the actual outcome of policies. An indication of the enormous variations can be found in statistics regarding dependency in the population. For example, in a recent study, figures given for full dependency among those 65 years of age and older range between 2% in Italy and 8.2% in France, those for partial dependency between 15% in the United Kingdom and 34% in the Netherlands (Pacolet, Bouten, Lanoye, Versieck 1999a). Standardised needs assessment combined with care plans might reduce room for discretion on the micro-level, in particular if this approach is accompanied by an improvement of data on long-term care issues. Overall, needs assessment plays an important role in the allocation of long-term care resources but long-term care policies are far from having a generally accepted definition of need and are far from using need as the only criterion for allocating long-term care in all the countries. (For an overview see Table 5.1.)

A second approach to allocate resources are *time-related principles*, in particular waiting-lists. Time related principles are used in long-term care either for practicality reasons, as an explicit or implicit concept of rationing or as an additional indicator of need. Waiting lists have been and still are an important explicit or implicit allocating principle in the residential care sector in most of the countries, although systematic evaluation is missing. Trends to support domiciliary care, economic restrictions for the further expansion of the residential care sector, and targeting of this sector towards the severely disabled, have more recently reduced the number of people on waiting lists (Rostgaard, Fridberg 1998; Rudda 1998).

Regarding waiting lists in the domiciliary care sector, there is evidence for waiting lists in the home help sector in the Netherlands, which is one of the driving forces for the development of independent providers outside the publicly financed scheme (Rostgaard, Fridberg 1998). In the four countries there is no legal right to receive home care, there is however such a guarantee for specific home nursing activities from the health system. But even here, procedures might be designed in a way that leads to considerable waiting time. In general, the existence of waiting lists is only a mediocre indicator for comparing unmet need across countries or even across local areas, as the demand for such services is very much determined by the existing supply structure.

Another form of time-related principles can be found in the Attendance Allowance scheme in the United Kingdom which requires that those applying must have been in need of care for at least six months.

The set of *status principles* includes a variety of principles such as age, family status, residence status or occupational status. In health and social care some of these principles are used as additional principles to define the target group. Age can be found in many payment for care programmes as an additional principle of allocating resources. Whereas the Austrian payment for care programme is open for disabled people of all age-groups, the Italian and partly the United Kingdom payment for care programmes differentiate according to age, but offer cash benefits for all age groups. In Italy there is a division between adults and those under the age of 18 but the actual allocation does not differ between these two age-groups. In the United Kingdom 65 years of age is the dividing line for receiving either Attendance Allowance or Disability Living Allowance, offering a different amount of benefits. Direct Payments in the United Kingdom are reserved to those between 18 and 65 years of age as well as elderly who entered the programme before they have reached the age of 65. But differentiation according to age can not only be found as an explicit principle. There also seem to exist hidden assumptions regarding different objectives in long-term care according to age. Long-term care related cash benefits differing according to age are just one example. Another example is the objective of independent living often identified as an objective with the interests of younger disabled people (Priestley 1999; Morris 1993).

As it has already been mentioned, in Italy and in Austria, and increasingly in the United Kingdom and in the Netherlands, informal care-giving resources are taken into account in the decision over the care arrangement. Hence, family status as well as the question of whether a person is living alone or together with other people, are used as criteria for allocating long-term care resources.

One of the principles to be found in all the countries is a rather high level of decentralisation, allowing considerable local variations – and hence differentiation according to residence status – in the provision of long-term care. Among the four countries under consideration, the Netherlands is the exception in this respect as there are important national standards alongside the organisation on the local level. Whereas this is seen as a major reason for a lack of co-ordination and a lack of flexibility in the Netherlands (Coolen, Weekers 1998), the opposite – shifting responsibilities to local authorities – is criticised for creating considerable inequalities across the country in the United Kingdom (Glendinning 1998; Walker 1995). Recent policy developments are aimed at a combination of the advantages of central and decentral policy making. Steps in this direction are nationwide payment for care programmes, the reservation of central public money for specific use, as well as national quality standards or guidelines.

Table 5.2 Means-related principles in allocating resources

	Austria	Italy	Netherlands	United Kingdom
Nursing homes	if financial means of those in need of care (including cash benefits) are not sufficient, costs will be covered by local authorities; they may be recovered from close family members	if financial means of those in need of care (including cash benefits) are not sufficient, costs will be covered by local authorities; they may be recovered from close family members	income-related co-payments from residents	if financial means of those in need of care (including cash benefits) are not sufficient, costs will be covered by local authorities; no legal obligation of maintenance for family members
Social services	co-payments differing across the country and across providers with regard to extent and means-testing; co-payments account for approx. 20-30% of total costs	co-payments differing across the country and across providers with regard to extent and means-testing; co-payments account for approx. 50% of total costs	co-payments related to household income and household composition; co-payments account for approx. 10-15% of total costs	co-payments differing across the country and across providers with regard to extent and means-testing; co-payments account for approx. 10-15% of total costs
Payments for care	not means-tested	not means-tested	income-related co-payments are deducted from the Personal Budget	cash benefits partly means-tested, partly not means-tested

Economic or *means-related principles* are increasingly important in allocating resources in long-term care (for an overview see Table 5.2). Means-testing is either used to allocate benefits in kind or in cash to those whose ability-to-pay is below a certain level or to design co-payments according to the ability-to-pay. In general, the ability-to-pay is based on the income of the client, but might be broadened covering assets as well as income and savings from close relatives. Financing residential care in Austria and Italy as well as in the United Kingdom is, first of all, based on the financial means of the clients including welfare benefits such as payments for care or Income Support in the United Kingdom. Total costs not covered will then be paid by local authorities. These costs might be recovered from close relatives in Austria and Italy, although there is much room for discretion in this respect. In the Netherlands, residential care is financed out of public funds with income-related co-payments from residents.

As a general rule, domiciliary services are covered by a combination of public funds and increasingly means-tested co-payments. Although these co-payments differ considerably within countries, rates tend to be lower in the Netherlands and in the United Kingdom and higher in Italy (see Table 5.2). Home nursing is offered free of charge in the United Kingdom and in Austria (with rather strict eligibility criteria). Otherwise, co-payments range between about 10-15% in the United Kingdom and in the Netherlands, as high as 20-30% in Austria and about 50% in Italy.

Payments for care are not means-tested in Austria and in Italy, except for payment for care programmes more recently introduced in Italy in some of the regions or municipalities. This is also true for some benefits in the United Kingdom (such as the Attendance Allowance and the Disability Living Allowance scheme), but there are means-tested programmes as well (such as the Carer Premium). In the personal budget programme in the Netherlands income related co-payments are deducted. Overall, payment for care programmes are a more or less important contribution to cover long-term care expenses. Covering an extended amount of care by external providers remains a privilege for those with private financial means to cover additional costs.

Apart from the distribution of burdens in the finance of long-term care, these economic principles have important implications on the provision of care. With the introduction of co-payments, economic constraints may lead to a reduction in the consumption of the respective services, in particular in low income groups. For this reason, co-payment models increasingly include means-testing in order to avoid negative consequences for the low-income groups regarding the consumption of professional services.

Another type of economic principles applies, if different forms of providing care result (or are supposed to result) in the same outcome. Here, efficiency could be used as an appropriate principle to decide which form of provision to promote. Although the outcome of caring in acute hospitals, in residential care settings or in the community will not be exactly the same, there is room for allocating resources among these different institutions according to the efficiency principle. And indeed, this is one of the driving forces for the redesign of long-term care systems in many countries. One example for an explicit approach in this direction can be found in the 7% rule in the Netherlands restricting the number of beds in the residential care sector. Similar explicit incentives are used to shift the actual provision from public providers to providers in the independent sector in the United Kingdom. Budgets are increasingly used as an instrument of guiding allocation. Apart from the examples already mentioned (reserving parts of the budget for specific purposes), overall limited budgets given to local authorities have a similar effect in that it puts pressure on these authorities to search for cost-effective ways for providing long-term care.

Obviously, most of the principles described are not used as single principles, but as *mixed principles*. The concept of need is combined with time-related principles, a variety of status principles, economic principles as well as *implicit principles*. In this latter case allocation of resources is (partly) determined by principles that are not explicitly stated in any regulation or guideline.

If people in need of care have to make out-of-pocket payments to get access to social services, this might to some extent exclude the poorest because of lack of purchasing power. This is even true if there is means-testing, as means-testing might involve consequences (e.g. stigmatisation) that create an incentive not to claim for a benefit. Attitudes towards care-giving, such as viewing external care as pushing off a moral obligation, may create incentives to offer informal care, even if there are formal services available. Such incentives seem to highly correlate with legal obligations to be found in the different countries and the amount of services offered in the formal sector.

The informational background of users might become an implicit principle favouring those with better access to information. For example, take-up ratios for cash benefits are often higher among those supported by social services as these also have an important role as providers of information. Other implicit principles in the allocation of resources might occur because of orientations of individual decision-makers, lobbying or political power. Considerable local variations in take-up ratios in the Italian payment for care programme seem to result to some extent from such implicit principles. In the United Kingdom, decentralised decision-making was introduced as an approach of effective and efficient coverage of needs under restricted financial resources. As shown before, evidence regarding the outcome of care management experiences is mixed.

There is a range of responses to negative effects arising from discretionary decision-making and implicit principles. One approach is to establish national standards aimed at guaranteeing equality in access and use of services or benefits and quality of long-term care services. This, however, tends to reduce flexibility, as partly seen from the Netherlands experience (Coolen, Weekers 1998). National standards in payment for care programmes are more definite in Austria, whereas in Italy, despite such standards, there are considerable variations across the country. In addition, the creation and support of lobbying associations, in particular the Carers Association in the United Kingdom, as well as improved information of care receivers and carers are steps to reduce inequalities arising from lack of information or lack of access to information.

Although the legal obligation to care for family members and the role of the family in society still very much shapes long-term care in Italy and in Austria, room for discretion is also used in these countries to reduce financial burdens in case of residential care. On the other hand, in the United Kingdom there is no such legal obligation. But, because of strict budget control, hidden assumptions about family obligations and increasing expectations regarding the potential role of the family seems to become more important in the assessment of care needs (Millar, Warman 1996).

Summary

The results with regard to what resources in long-term care are allocated by welfare state policies according to which principles may be summarised as follows: The division between private and public responsibilities and the level of in-kind services provided shows a clear hierarchy ranging from the Netherlands with a high level of public responsibility, a broad range of services and a high number of people using services in the residential as well as in the domiciliary care sector, to Italy with a low level of public responsibility and a low level of service supply from the welfare state. Austria and the United Kingdom are situated between the other two countries, with Austria, in terms of in-kind benefits, closer to Italy. Whereas in-kind provision is emphasised the most in the Netherlands, payment for care programmes are an additional approach in the other countries, which is rather important in Austria. Choice in alternatives is increased between residential, semi-residential and domiciliary care as well as between formal and informal care-giving, but restricted by more rigid standardised needs assessment and co-payments becoming more widespread in all four countries.

Need is in the centre of the allocation principles, but all the countries are far from allocating resources just according to an interpretation of need that is related to health condition and resulting requirements for care. In this respect all the countries are far from realising an equity concept of 'equal care for equal needs'. What can be observed in all countries investigated is a tendency towards stricter needs assessment. The public response to long-term care needs is restricting residential care more and more to those with severe disabilities, and domiciliary care to home nursing and personal care. As responsibilities in long-term care within the public sector are very much on regional and local levels, the allocation of resources is characterised by considerable local variations. The exception are the Netherlands where national regulation is strongest. Overall, means-testing and income-related co-payments are becoming more important in the in-kind service sector in all the countries. These measures are aimed at cost-containment, providing more cost-effective care, and sharing financial responsibilities. In the residential care sector, means-testing in Austria and in Italy includes not just those in need of care but close family members too. On the other hand, in these two countries the existing payment for care programmes are not means-tested.

5.2 Equity choices in the finance of long-term care

Different from provision, the finance of long-term care on the macro-level is mainly the responsibility of central public bodies, even if local authorities do have room to levy their own taxes in some countries. Apart from public finance via taxes and social insurance contributions as well as out-of-pocket payments, long-term care is to a considerable extent financed on the basis of informal care-giving without direct compensation. Whereas allocation of burdens through taxes and social insurance contributions is based on explicit principles, the extent to which these taxes and insurance contributions are dedicated explicitly for long-term care issues – that is to what extent they are earmarked – is limited. An overview to the structure of taxes and social insurance contributions in Austria, Italy, the Netherlands and the United Kingdom is given in Table 5.3. Overall, tax receipts range between 41.9% and 44.4% of GDP in Austria, Italy and the Netherlands, and 35.4% of GDP in the United Kingdom.

Moving towards the private sector, and even more moving towards the informal sector, explicit principles become less and less important. Nevertheless, there is a wide range of incentives creating implicit principles for a specific distribution of burdens in financing long-term care.

Table 5.3 Tax structure (including social security contributions) in Austria, Italy, the Netherlands and the United Kingdom

	A	I	NL	UK
Total tax receipts (% of GDP; 1997)	44.3	44.4	41.9	35.4
Tax structure (as % of total tax receipts; 1997)				
Personal income tax	22.1	25.3	15.6	24.8
Corporate income tax	4.7	9.5	10.5	12.1
Social security contributions – employees	14.2	6.6	26.5	7.5
Social security contributions – employers	16.8	23.5	6.2	9.6
Taxes on goods and services	28.2	25.9	28.0	35.0
Other taxes	14.0	9.2	13.2	11.0

Source: OECD (2000)

The following discussion attempts to analyse equity approaches in financing long-term care in Austria, Italy, the Netherlands and the United Kingdom. In this chapter it will be investigated what burdens are allocated in long-term care policies and what principles are used in the design of allocation. As with the provision of long-term care the focus is on explicit and implicit public choices with particular respect to be paid to the role of informal care givers as in-kind financiers of long-term care. A discussion of these choices with regard to equity objectives will follow in chapter 5.3.

What burdens?

The *burdens to be shared* in the finance of long-term care are the means to finance long-term care in order to provide resources for the actual care. It includes the finance of residential care, domiciliary care, payment for care programmes as well as overheads. In addition, care is offered informally without direct compensation. Although there is no raising of funds in this case, informal care-giving does of course produce considerable opportunity costs.

The use of the various options to finance long-term care in Austria, Italy, the Netherlands and the United Kingdom is shown in Table 5.4. Compared to health care, *tax-financed* models dominate over *social insurance* models in long-term care. Although the insurance model tends to be a major issue in many of the discussions on the future finance of long-term care, Germany and to less extent Luxembourg are the only examples in Europe where this in fact is the main source of publicly financing long-term care. In most other countries, including those covered by this study, finance is primarily tax-based and just to a smaller extent based on social insurance contributions (see Table 5.4).

Private insurance plays a minor role in all of the countries. Although there is some trend towards an increase in such insurance policies, the overall importance is still very much restricted. The US as well as the Europe experiences suggest that this minor role occurs even in a situation where public support is rather limited and family involvement in financial terms is potentially considerable (e.g. Pauly 1990; Hennessy 1997; chapter 2.4).

Table 5.4 Financing long-term care in Austria, Italy, the Netherlands and the United Kingdom

Country	Taxation	Social Insurance	Private Insurance	Out-of-pocket Payments	Informal Care-Giving
Austria	dominant form of public finance	for medical nursing care	very limited	in particular for residential care, increasingly for domiciliary care	legal obligation for family care
Italy	dominant form of public finance	for health-related expenditure	very limited	in particular for residential care, increasingly for domiciliary care	legal obligation for family care
Netherlands	dominant form of public finance via AWBZ based on taxes as well as social insurance contributions		very limited	co-payments for residential care as well as domiciliary care	division of state and private responsibilities
United Kingdom	mainly central government taxes, plus some social insurance contributions and local taxes		very limited	in particular for residential care, co-payments for domiciliary care	no legal obligation, but increasing requirement of private solutions

Source: chapter 4.3

Out-of-pocket payments do play an important role in all of the countries in the form of purely private consumption as well as co-payments. Purely private consumption either means that with specific goods or services there is no form of public support at all, or that individuals prefer a private solution over a solution that involves public subsidies. Typical examples for privately financed resources are specific aids, dietary requirements, travel costs, etc. Other examples are places in residential care settings or domiciliary care outside the publicly (co-)financed sector. In the Netherlands, a reduction of home help provided by the public sector as well as waiting lists in this sector, lead to an increasing importance of private providers. In the United Kingdom clients are offered to opt for a more expensive residential care setting, than the one chosen by the assessment team, if they are willing to top up the fee.

In recent years, an increase in *co-payments* can be observed across all countries, even if for different reasons. The introduction of out-of-pocket payments in the nursing home sector does not only offer an additional source of finance, but also works as an economic incentive by changing the economic 'attractiveness' of residential versus domiciliary care. In Italy the health aspect in residential care settings is covered by the regions. Otherwise clients have to pay for residential care settings with the public sector coming in again according to the social assistance principle if means are not sufficient. In Austria as well as in the United Kingdom, income, savings and welfare benefits (payments for care in Austria and Income Support and other benefits in the United Kingdom) have to be used. If these sources do not cover the costs of residential care, the provinces or the local authorities cover the rest, which might be recovered from close family members in Austria. In the Netherlands user fees, which are increasingly means-tested, are a supplement to the finance via AWBZ.

In the social service sector, out-of-pocket payments are also used as a means to finance such services as well as to guide the consumption of services. And co-payments become more widespread in the social service sector. For Italy it is estimated that about 50% of social services are paid out-of-pocket. In the Netherlands social services are financed from AWBZ with co-payments and/or membership fees from clients. In the United Kingdom nursing home care is the only service that is offered free of charge, whereas for home help financed through local funds, co-payments have to be made. In Austria, the introduction of the payment for care programme providing cash benefits to care receivers was followed – in at least some provinces – by a considerable increase in co-payments to be made by clients.

Finally, the finance of long-term care is based on *informal care-giving* without direct compensation. As has been shown earlier (chapter 2.1), this is the dominant form of providing and financing long-term care even in those countries where service delivery reaches a quite high level, as for example in the Netherlands. The role of families in long-term care provision and financing becomes obvious not just in the empirical observation but is made explicit by legal regulation in Italy and in Austria, where family members are legally obliged to contribute to 'maintenance'. There is, however, room for discretion with respect to lowering this obligation in both countries. An increase of family obligations can be observed in the United Kingdom and in the Netherlands although there is no 'legal' obligation to provide or finance long-term care. In the United Kingdom, the assessment of care needs increasingly includes an assessment of the availability of kin as care givers. Evidence shows that the number of hours spent by professionals for domestic care in the United Kingdom and in the Netherlands has been dropping considerably, shifting burdens of financing domestic care towards the formal and informal private sector (Rostgaard, Fridberg 1998).

In parts of Austria and parts of Italy, informal care-giving is often the only choice for organising care for relatives – except for a limited number of people which are cared for in residential care settings. And in parts of the population in these two countries there are strong attitudes regarding long-term care as a family obligation. However, variations within the countries are considerable with a general tendency towards an increasing importance of professional services and changing attitudes towards 'accepting' the consumption of such services. In the other countries, in particular in the Netherlands, the overall level of informal care-giving is lower, but still the main source of care-giving.

In all the countries there is an increasing awareness of the role of the informal sector. The informal sector has always been the major 'financier' of long-term care, with the major actual burden on spouses or other close female family members. In those countries with a comparatively higher level of social service support there even is a re-increase of private informal help (Szebehely cit. in Eliasson Lappalainen, Nilsson Motevasel 1997). There also is, however, an increased awareness of the role of informal care-giving. The awareness is growing for two very different reasons. First of all, informal care-giving becomes increasingly important because of financial constraints and related tendencies to limit public responsibilities. Secondly, there is a slow growing awareness of the enormous burdens associated with informal care-giving ranging from disadvantages in the formal labour market and in social protection systems to negative effects on social integration and on the health of carers. Recent approaches to explicitly support informal care-giving include payment for care programmes, the recognition of informal work in social insurance schemes as well as respite care (Bettio, Prechal 1998). An increased recognition of informal care in the policy process in the United Kingdom and in the Netherlands arises from the establishment of carers associations. Overall, respective attempts are still very limited regarding coverage and extent. In addition, recent developments – as for example strengthening the labour market link of welfare benefits – tend to further increase opportunity costs of informal care-giving.

Among whom?

The units among whom burdens might be shared are *individuals*, *families*, *households*, *companies* as well as *political units*. Whereas the question of who has to actually pay specific taxes or contributions in monetary terms is rather explicit, the question of incidence, that is the identification of the unit that finally has to bear the burden, is far from clear (see chapter 3.5).

For taxes and social insurance contributions the identification of the focal unit becomes even more difficult as there is no specific earmarking for most long-term care funds. Incidence, therefore, is a result of the incidence of specific sources, such as income taxes, property taxes or social insurance contributions. Although there is earmarking with social insurance contributions, this tends to refer just to health care, or health and social care in general. For example, AWBZ funds in the Netherlands apart from covering long-term care issues, also include long-term admissions to hospitals or institutionalised psychiatric care.

Because of this complexity empirical research tends to use standard incidence assumptions, according to which – as one standard assumption – personal income and property taxes have to be borne by taxpayers, corporate income taxes by shareholders, and employee and employer insurance contributions by employees (see e.g. van Doorslaer, Wagstaff 1993).

Out-of-pocket payments including co-payments will be made either by the individual in need of care, or – as far as long-term care is regarded as a broader family obligation – by other family members. The fact that families are a major focal unit not just in the provision but also in the finance of long-term care becomes even more obvious in the actual informal provision of long-term care without direct compensation. As described in chapter 2.1 the bulk of care-giving, and hence the bulk of opportunity costs, tends to be borne by one close family member, dominantly by spouses, daughters and daughters-in-law. The actual distribution follows a variety of social, financial or cultural determinants to be found inside and outside the family. An explicit obligation of specific family members exists with the legal obligation of maintenance in Italy and in Austria, which becomes relevant if residents in nursing homes or residential homes are unable to fully cover fees.

How?

The allocation of burdens in the finance of long long-term care is based on economic principles, status principles, mixed principles and a wide range of implicit principles. Compared to the allocation of resources in the provision of care, there is not much room for implicit principles in the public sector raising funds for long-term care through taxes and social insurance contributions, whereas such implicit principles become increasingly important with moving towards the informal sector and decreasing public regulation and standard-setting.

First of all, *economic* or *means-related principles* are used in raising public funds through taxes and social insurance contributions. Except for the Netherlands, most of the public long-term care funds are tax-based. Personal income related tax systems are designed as progressive systems, that is taxes of lower income groups represent a smaller proportion of their income as with middle or higher income groups. Most other taxes are proportionate or even regressive, as for example most indirect taxes like the value-added tax.

Social insurance contributions tend to be regressive in an overall perspective, as there usually is an earning ceiling above which no additional contributions have to be paid. Below this earning ceiling contributions are, in general, proportionate. Proportionality may, however, be restricted, if those with low earnings are exempt or if social insurance contributions differ across professions. The latter case is one of the reasons why empirical evidence shows that the former Italian health insurance system was progressive (Paci, Wagstaff 1993).

Out-of-pocket payments, co-payments and means-testing are quite common in the design of long-term care systems. Financing residential care in Austria and Italy as well as in the United Kingdom is primarily based on clients' financial means including benefits such as payments for care, or Income Support in the United Kingdom. In Italy, the health aspect of caring for people in nursing homes is covered by the regions. Total costs not covered herewith will then be financed by local authorities. These costs might be recovered from close relatives in Austria and Italy, although there is much room for discretion in this respect. In the Netherlands residential care – residential homes are in a transition period – is financed out of public funds with co-payments from residents which are related to income.

Hence, in all the countries income and assets (except for the Netherlands) are used as criteria for the allocation of burdens. The contribution by people in need of care and their families in Austria and in Italy is following social assistance principles and might be considerable, the more so as there is a legal obligation of maintenance between family members in the case of long-term care needs. This does not exist in the Netherlands and in the United Kingdom. The financial burden on residents and their families has been lowered in recent years with the introduction of universal payment for care programmes, in particular in Austria. In the Netherlands, co-payments in the residential care sector are limited to an income-related payment. Another economic principle in the residential care sector is used in the United Kingdom: If local authorities have to finance residential care because individual financial resources do not cover full cost, these authorities choose the residential care setting. Relatives, however, have the opportunity to opt for another nursing or residential home, if they are willing to top up the fee in that residential care setting.

Domiciliary services are covered by a combination of public funds and increasingly means-tested co-payments. Although these co-payments differ considerably within countries, they tend to be lower in the Netherlands and higher in Italy. In the Netherlands means-tested co-payments and/or membership fees have to be paid by the clients. In the United Kingdom co-payment regulations increasingly use means-tested co-payments instead of flat-rate co-payments. Nursing care is still fully covered by central public money. Another form of co-payment is to be found in the personal budget programme in the Netherlands, where income related co-payments are deducted.

Apart from co-payments, out-of-pocket payments are made to buy services in the formal private sector at full cost. To the extent to which there is no public intervention in the private residential or domiciliary care sector, coverage of care needs by residential or domiciliary care services in the formal private sector remains a privilege of higher income groups.

Family status is the most important *status principle* in allocating burdens. In Italy and in Austria there is a legal obligation to care for family members, which in Italy includes the extended family, in Austria spouses, parents and children. The legal obligation gives no definition of what sort support has to be, and in reality there is considerable room for discretion in the enforcement of this obligation. Apart from the actual distribution of covering long-term care needs between family and the state, family obligations become most obvious in the case of residential care. Here, in both countries income from family members might be used to cover costs of residence. If financial means from clients are not sufficient, the remaining amount is covered by the public sector out of social assistance funds, which may be recovered from family members. Another type of status principles is occupational status, as to be found in tax and even more in social insurance systems with contributions differing accordingly.

Implicit principles become more important the more the informal sector becomes the major financier of long-term care. A legal obligation of maintenance between family members does exist in Austria and in Italy, where the amount of family care-giving is larger than in the United Kingdom or in the Netherlands. But even in these latter countries, informal long-term care covers the bulk of long-term care-giving. Regarding the explicit or implicit intervention through public policies – apart from the legal obligation just mentioned – different scenarios have to be distinguished as will be discussed below.

Without state intervention and due to economic burdens arising from long-term care needs that can not be fully covered in a formal private market by any average income earner, it is very likely that families, households or other informal networks offer care-giving. Whether and to what extent informal care-giving actually is offered is among other issues determined by values and attitudes towards family obligations, which in turn are also determined by the role of the welfare state. Family obligations are still quite strong in Europe, although there are considerable north-south differences in this respect. Family obligations as perceived in the population are much stronger in central-western and southern Europe than in the Nordic countries. On the other hand, it is in these countries where people most expect a reduction in the availability of informal care (Walker, Maltby 1997). Opportunity costs for single main care givers tend to be considerable and include forgone wages, disadvantages regarding the position in the labour market and career opportunities as well as disadvantages in the social security system (see e.g. Carmichael, Charles 1998; White-Means 1997). And there are considerable negative effects on the health status of informal carers, the involvement in social life as well as on family relationships (see e.g. Mengani, Lamura, Melchiorre 1999; RIS MRC CTAS 1998; Aldridge, Becker 1996; Badelt, Holzmann-Jenkins, Matul, Österle 1997).

Apart from a basic 'no intervention' model, the state intervenes in informal care-giving in a number of different ways, either promoting or discouraging informal care-giving. Informal long-term care-giving is increasingly supported through payment for care programmes, existing in Austria, Italy, the United Kingdom and to very little extent in the Netherlands. Payments are directed to care receivers in Austria and in Italy (with the opportunity to transfer these benefits to informal care givers). In the United Kingdom there are also payments directed to informal care givers. Such payments can be seen as a recognition of the work undertaken in the informal sector as well as a contribution to real and/or opportunity costs arising with informal care-giving. If such payments lead to a reduction of full-time to part-time employment or even a resignation from formal employment, they could even increase overall opportunity costs that are borne by informal care givers.

Leave-programmes as well as the recognition of informal care-giving in the social security system are additional approaches to reduce opportunity costs. As existing leave-programmes are just offering short-term leaves, they are designed for short-term care, such as illnesses or terminal care, but not for long-term care obligations. An exception are medium-term leaves to be found in some collective arrangements in the Netherlands and in Italy. (Bettio, Prechal 1998) The recognition of informal care-giving in social security schemes might considerably lower the opportunity cost of informal care-giving. Other opportunity costs arising from reducing formal employment such as difficulties in re-entering the labour market or with career opportunities, are not affected.

On the other hand, public choices might also discourage informal care-giving. Such an effect occurs if social security is strictly connected to formal employment or if earning levels make double income an economic necessity. By such measures, opportunity costs of informal work further increase. It might become economically impossible to reduce formal employment or to resign from the formal labour market. Due to existing levels of services provided this tends not to result in a considerably smaller amount of informal care-giving, but in the necessity to organise informal care-giving alongside work and herewith creating a double burden. This, of course, is much more of an issue in those countries where the extent of formal services is lower, as in Austria and in Italy. But even in countries like the Netherlands or the Nordic countries, enormous burdens are left to the informal sector.

Summary

Reflecting the role of the state in long-term care, public finance is most important in the Netherlands, followed by the United Kingdom and Austria, and least important in Italy. Out-of-pocket payments do play an important role in all the countries, and recent changes in the long-term care systems have even reinforced the co-payment approach. Apart from out-of-pocket payments in the purely private sector, out-of-pocket payments are a major source of finance in the residential care sector in Austria, Italy and the

United Kingdom. Although there are considerable variations within each of the countries, co-payments have to be made in the domiciliary care sector in all the countries. And finally, informal long-term care remains a most important source of financing long-term care in all the countries, most importantly in Austria and Italy.

In Table 5.5 the distribution of burdens to finance long-term care in nursing homes and in the domiciliary sector is given. Because of problems in definition and availability of reliable data, figures have to be dealt with caution, they do however offer a good picture of the basic trends to be observed. Financing through public authorities is highest in the Netherlands, considerably lower in Austria and even more so in Italy. In addition, in Italy the distribution of burdens varies considerably between regions and local authorities (Gori 2001).

Table 5.5 Financing nursing homes, home help and home nursing (% of overall costs; average)

	nursing homes			home help / home nursing		
	private [1]	public	other [2]	private [1]	public	other [2]
Austria	20-30	60	10	20-30	60-70	5
Italy	considerable local variations			considerable local variations		
Netherlands	11	89	0	- / 14	81 / 86	- / 0
United Kingdom	30	70	0	9 / 0	91 / 100	0 / 0

- ... indicates missing data.
1) private: the person in need of care or relatives.
2) other: private insurance, sponsors, charities.

Source: Pacolet, Bouten, Lanoye, Versieck (1999a)

As for the principles used in allocating burdens, means-related principles, as defined in part 3, dominate. They are used to design tax and social insurance systems as well as co-payment systems.

For the Netherlands, AWBZ contributions are progressive at low income levels, but regressive at higher income levels. Personal income tax is progressive, this however counts for a considerably smaller proportion of the payments. Overall, the tax and social contributions system in the Netherlands is regressive (van Doorslaer, Wagstaff, Janssen 1993). The same is true for Italy, where health specific payments are reported to be progressive at low income levels, but regressive at high income levels.

Against a general assumption, in Italy progressivity has been measured even in the social insurance system which most probably is caused by varying contributions of different professional groups and their position in the income distribution (Paci, Wagstaff 1993). For the United Kingdom the finance of health care is reported as almost proportionate with a progressive income tax system (O'Donnell, Propper, Upward 1993). Similar results are reported for Austria (the self-employed excluded) (WIFO 1996). Whereas (in a household perspective) direct taxes are progressive, indirect taxes as well as social insurance contributions are regressive, resulting in an overall almost proportionate taxes and contributions system. Long-term care in Austria is mainly tax-financed – apart from medical nursing care which is covered by the social health insurance system, but represents only a small proportion of total long-term care expenditure. Hence, financing long-term care in Austria through taxes and social insurance contributions tends to be proportionate or just slightly progressive.

Although calculations reported mainly refer to the health care system, they can be used as an indicator for financing long-term care. For the Netherlands and the United Kingdom, financing is similar to health care to the extent that long-term care is financed through taxes and social insurance contributions. There tends to be more progressivity in the Austrian and in the Italian long-term system compared to the health care system because public finance of long-term care is based on taxes rather than social insurance contributions in these countries.

In systems with universal or almost universal public coverage of health risks, private insurance contributions tend to be progressive. This is because in these systems higher income groups tend to have more private insurance coverage than middle or low income groups. Although many countries are far from offering universal public coverage against long-term care risks, private insurance solutions in long-term care are very limited. In existing private long-term care insurance markets, contributions tend to be quite high and, hence, just affordable for high income groups.

Out-of-pocket payments tend to be highly regressive in health care (van Doorslaer, Wagstaff, Rutten 1993). It might be assumed that this is the same in long-term care, the more so as there usually is a ceiling for such co-payments. The exception is the low-income groups, if they are exempted from co-payments. On the other hand out-of-pocket payments to buy services on the formal for-profit market tend to be progressive for reasons given with private insurance contributions.

Quantitative information pertaining to the informal care sector is very limited. Evidence of the determinants of informal care-giving (e.g. Finch 1989) and the relationship between informal carers and formal service provision (Twigg, Atkin 1995) identifies a series of factors determining kind, extent and distribution of informal care-giving. These factors include attitudes towards informal care-giving and the role of family by carers, the person cared-for as well as other family members, and determinants of intra-family relationships such as altruism, reciprocity, or autonomy.

In addition, the actual decision whether and to what extent to provide informal care is determined by a number of structural variables (see e.g. Klein 1996; Rhoades 1998; Twigg, Atkin 1995; Kemper 1992). Co-residence tends to be an important indicator of the amount of informal care-giving, with a considerable higher amount of actual care offered in the case of co-residence. With higher income levels there tends to be more consumption of formal services and a lower level of informal care-giving. The dominant forms of care-giving are between spouses, care for the elderly generation by daughters and daughters-in-law, and caring for children (other than parenting). Women tend to be much more involved in informal care-giving, which is particularly true for informal care for the parents generation. Empirical evidence shows that formal employment plays a minor role in determining the decision whether or not to offer informal care-giving, although formal employment commitments tend to be lowered in the case of severe and long-lasting care needs (see chapter 2.1). But disregarding the implications of formal employment alongside informal care-giving obligations would be completely misleading. Formal employment offers social security rights and regular income. Informal care-giving alongside formal employment commitments means a large additional burden for the respective person and, in the case of lowering formal employment, long-term disadvantages with regard to the social and economic situation of the care giver (social security rights, career opportunities, social integration, health, etc.). With regard to opportunity costs related to labour market and social security, these predominantly affect women.

Regarding distributional consequences, this results in considerably higher burdens on women, the more so as they tend to be care givers in their working-age, whereas men tend to be care givers when they are retired. From the 'ability-to-pay' perspective women in lower income groups tend to spend more hours on informal care-giving, which represents an extremely regressive system, which, however, to some extent is outweighed by the fact that those in the higher income-levels spend more on formal social services.

5.3 Equity choices and equity objectives in European long-term care systems

Choices made in public policies with regard to the object (what?), the subject (whom?) and the principles of allocation (how?) are shaping equity approaches in the welfare state. These have been comparatively investigated for the provision and the finance of long-term care in Austria, Italy, the Netherlands and the United Kingdom. It will now be examined whether or not and to what extent these choices fit with basic equity objectives. As discussed in part 3 and in chapter 4.2, the study takes a set of equity objectives, reflecting different ideas about equity in the welfare state, as the reference point. By following this approach it acknowledges the diversity and complexity of potential equity choices and equity objectives. The set of equity objectives identified in chapter 4.2 consists of the following elements: guaranteeing minimum standards to reduce and/or to prevent absolute poverty, supporting living standards to reduce and/or to prevent large drops in the living standard, reducing inequalities (horizontally and vertically) and social integration by enhancing personal autonomy and equalising social rights and responsibilities. A brief overview to what extent these objectives are promoted in the four countries with respect to those in need of care and informal care givers is given in Tables 5.6 and 5.7, respectively, presented at the end of chapter 5.3.

All the countries in question are offering social policy schemes providing some *minimum level* of economic resources. Whereas in many social policy areas this is just a second pillar in the respective welfare states, instruments going beyond prevention or reduction of poverty in case of long-lasting severe long-term care needs still do not exist in many countries or have been introduced only recently. Looking at the countries under consideration in this study, the minimum standard objective is strongest in Italy and in Austria. In both these countries, residential care is financed out of income, savings and welfare benefits of the person in need of care. This is also true for the United Kingdom. If these financial means are not sufficient to cover full costs, the difference is paid by local authorities or regions. In Italy and Austria this can be recovered from close family members. The situation is different in the case of domiciliary care, where clients' co-payments are smaller and limited to a means-tested component.

Payment for care programmes are offering a substantial amount of relief, in particular in Austria where payments are not means-tested and where the benefit rate is considerably higher than in other countries. Hence, the risk of becoming absolutely poor is reduced. It does, however, not necessarily prevent people from becoming absolutely poor in the case of residential care, because fees for residences are considerably higher than payment for care rates and even the maximum rate of the allowance plus an average pension does not cover full costs. In Italy, allowances are smaller, characterised by local variations and, hence, offer a much smaller intervention to reduce or to prevent poverty. In the United Kingdom, the risk of becoming poor is limited as costs of residential care covered by local authorities are not recovered from close family members. More recently, however, there is an increasing recognition of kin as potential care givers in the assessment procedure, which can be seen as an implicit approach to shift responsibilities to families. Overall, it is just the Netherlands where public long-term care policies are clearly and generally going beyond the minimum standard objective.

Public finance within tax or social insurance systems is protecting a minimum standard and with regard to equity concerns, going beyond that objective. What remains is informal long-term care-giving as in-kind finance of care. With regard to equity objectives, the recognition of informal long-term care is very limited. The actual distribution of burdens remains in the private informal sphere, shifting opportunity costs to informal carers most of whom are women. In a situation of limited support or relief by social services, or if residences are – financially or technically – not available, the informal carers are put in a precarious situation, even more so for carers in their working age. Care-giving obligations hinder formal employment, future career opportunities and the inclusion in social protection systems. Payment for care programmes in Austria, Italy and the United Kingdom offer some relief if payments are transferred to care givers. Payments for care to care givers in the United Kingdom are designed as a premium to Income Support and, hence, explicitly designed as a measure to prevent absolute poverty. Measures to include informal care givers in the social protection system are a step to reduce opportunity costs arising from informal care giving. But respective measures are very much limited in all the countries. Existing leave programmes are just short-term and are not an effective tool to support long-term care givers. Apart from very modest attempts to support informal care-giving, there also have been explicit measures reinforcing informal care-giving obligations by recognising the potential of family care-giving in needs assessment in the United Kingdom or by reducing the amount of care offered as public support in the United Kingdom and in the Netherlands.

Supporting living standards aims at the reduction or prevention of large drops in the individual living situation. Generally, this is achieved by supporting people in case long-term care needs occur. In the care systems under consideration, a deterioration in the living standard is avoided to the extent to which payments are made or services are provided free of charge. This might be achieved through direct provision, purchasing provision, or insurance systems. Overall, compared to related policy fields such as health or pensions, being in need of long-term care means a considerably higher risk of dropping in the standard of living. Support in this respect is highest in the Netherlands. Residential as well as domiciliary care services are most developed in this country and co-payments by clients are limited to means-related contributions. Support by these institutional settings is considerably lower in the other countries, particularly in Italy where these settings do not even exist in parts of the country. If formal services are used, drops in the living standard may arise when co-payments or out-of-pocket payments are required. Such payments are important in the residential care sector in Italy, Austria and in the United Kingdom. In Austria and in Italy this obligation even includes close family members and, hence, extends the risk of dropping in the living standard. Large drops are less likely in the case of domiciliary care (if such services exist), but might still be significant in the case of severe and long-lasting care needs. On the other hand, it is in these countries where living standards are supported through cash benefits, in particular in Austria were payments are comparatively high covering a larger number of people in need of care.

Differences in the ability-to-pay are recognised in the design of tax and insurance systems. Whereas obligations to contribute to the finance of residential and domiciliary care settings have been discussed above, financing long-term care through informal care-giving remains again very much in the black box of intra-family allocations. The support of living-standards through welfare state policies is limited to those measures offering relief by formal care services or those measures aimed at informal care givers. This includes the recognition of care work in social protection systems and the provision of payments for care. Cash benefits however – by the majority of such programmes – are directed to care receivers. Regarding these measures, the risk of loosening in individual living standards is lowest in the Netherlands because of comparatively more extensive formal services with lower co-payments to be made by users, followed by the United Kingdom (with a combination of formal services and payments for care) and Austria (payments for care and increasingly social services in the community). Italy is characterised by enormous variations across the country, on average informal care givers are in a more precarious situation.

With regard to the objective of *redistribution*, vertical and horizontal aspects have to be distinguished. Horizontal equity addresses redistribution between the healthy and those in need of care. This objective is achieved to the extent to which people in need of care are supported by public policies. There is no full coverage of long-term care needs in any of the countries. Coverage through in-kind benefits is highest in the Netherlands followed by the United Kingdom. Coverage through cash benefits is highest in Austria and in the United Kingdom. To what extent horizontally equalising effects are achieved is not just decided through choosing specific need-related principles of allocation. Considerable horizontal inequalities may persist because of implicit principles and room for discretion in decentralised bodies of decision making. This causes – together with other factors – many territorial variations in all the countries, most of all in Italy, followed by Austria and the United Kingdom. In the Netherlands, because of much stricter national regulation, the inequalities are smaller. Differences are primarily found in the in-kind sector. In Italy and Austria this sector is characterised by decentralised responsibilities and enormous differences across the country. In the United Kingdom local variations are also a consequence of explicit measures to decentralise decision-making in community care. For cash benefits the picture is different. In the Austrian process of implementing the new payment for care programme following national guidelines for the assessment of needs, variations in take-up and in the needs-benefits relationship could be kept very small and even further reduced over time. In Italy, there are considerable differences in the actual take-up rate of payments for care. This constitutes inequalities across the country. As these inequalities are opposite to those in the in-kind sector, they partly balance – in an overall simplified perspective – inequalities in the two segments. Implicit principles do, however, not just refer to geographical inequalities, but also to inequalities between socio-economic groups. Evidence here is much more limited. It is, however, conceivable that a complex design of benefit schemes, such as with cash benefits in the UK, a lack of information and consumer power create such inequalities. For the United Kingdom, there is evidence of variations in take-up ratios among socio-economic groups (Department of Health 1998).

Vertical redistribution through long-term care systems is generally very small (see chapter 5.2). There are progressive effects to the extent to which public long-term care is financed through income taxes, which is more important in Austria, Italy and the United Kingdom. Other forms of financing long-term care are proportional or even regressive. This is true for financing long-term care through social insurance contributions in the Netherlands as well as most co-payment schemes. Any redistributive effects are restricted to the extent to which low-income groups are exempt from co-payments and/or to the extent to which such payments depend on the ability-to-pay.

Interventions in the sphere of informal care-giving for reasons of redistribution are limited to those measures discussed before, that is payments directed to informal carers, and the inclusion in social protection systems. To this extent horizontal redistribution occurs, rather limited overall. With recovering costs of long-term care from family members, potential inequalities are even extended to the family of those in need of care.

The discussion of *social integration* as an equity objective in chapter 4.2. leads to the identification of personal autonomy and social rights as the two corner stones to be addressed. The overall effects of the respective long-term care systems on issues of social integration can not be judged without taking the social and cultural background in these countries into account. What will be done here, is to discuss the implications of the policy approaches in the four countries on the two aspects, personal autonomy and social rights and responsibilities.

Personal autonomy defined as positive autonomy very much depends on the resource situation, covered by the three objectives discussed before. There is, however, at least one more major aspect that might be directly influenced by state policies, that is choice sets. Here, some similarities in qualitative trends (not in the extent) can be observed: All the countries investigated spend some efforts on a diversification of long-term care systems offering opportunities between the traditional approach of residential care or social services and informal care as well as measures to integrate the various services. (For an overview of trends in Europe see e.g. Pacolet, Bouten, Lanoye, Versieck 2000 or Giarchi 1996.) In terms of services provided, choice has been traditionally stronger in the Netherlands and in the United Kingdom compared to Austria and Italy and this still is the case. However, there have been measures to improve the situation in both of the latter countries, more so in Austria where there is a nationwide agreement to develop respective services until 2010. Whereas choice has been increased with regard to the service mix, access to specific services tends to be reduced by stricter assessment of needs taking into account the availability of informal care opportunities. This can be observed in the Netherlands as well as in the United Kingdom. In the Netherlands, public support in the case of nursing care or more severe long-term care needs is increased, but reduced for personal or domestic care. In the United Kingdom the possibility of family care is increasingly recognised in the assessment of needs. With regard to benefits in kind, availability in financial and technical terms as well as in diversity, and hence support of personal autonomy, is highest in the Netherlands and lowest in Italy.

A different approach to increase choice is offering cash benefits which allow recipients to freely choose how to use the money. This is realised in Austria and in Italy, and partly in cash payment programmes in the United Kingdom, whereas personal budgets in the Netherlands are very much restricted regarding their use. Cash benefits – apart from relieving the economic situation – will broaden choice sets, if alternatives are available. As shown this is not the case in parts of Italy and limited in parts of Austria. Here, however, cash programmes are an incentive for the development of such programmes as they are increasing the ability to contribute to the finance of professional or semi-professional services.

From the informal carers' point of view, personal autonomy requires that the person is free to choose whether to offer informal care or not. Here, just those aspects which might be directly influenced by state policies will be discussed, without neglecting most important factors in intra-family allocations and the role of the private sector. It has been repeatedly stressed that public support for informal care is limited in all four countries. There is an increase in choice sets because of a broader range of services available in all the countries. Choice sets have also been improved with the introduction of cash benefits. Although most of these programmes are directed at those in need of care, there are positive effects on informal care givers. Apart from an increase in the ability-to-pay (from a family or household perspective) the financial recognition of care work is emphasised. Though there is an increase in choice sets, there also have been effects that made the various choices more costly to informal care givers. These effects arise in particular from connecting welfare benefits and regular labour market participation as well as difficulties in combining care work and work in the regular labour market. Attempts to restrict access to residential care shifts more responsibility to informal care givers and restricts choice. This will either require care givers to withdraw from the regular labour market in case of long-lasting severe care-needs and limited support by social services or to combine care work and work in the regular labour market, in both cases loading immense burdens onto informal care givers. Altogether, the focus of social policies on extending personal autonomy of informal carers is still very narrow.

The objective of *promoting* and *equalising rights* (in the broader sense of *social rights*) includes the issues of rights instead of charity, dignity and the prevention of stigmatising or socially excluding effects. Long-term care is regarded as an issue of social rights. Historically, however, it has been an almost hidden agenda offering mainly social assistance. Only in the northern European countries and the UK has there been a tradition of long-term care as a social right going beyond the social assistance idea. At the same time, however, long-term care is also regarded as an issue with considerable private responsibility. Even in countries with broad public support, informal care is playing the dominant role in the provision and finance of long-term care. And indeed, recent policy attempts in many countries are even reducing public responsibilities in specific spheres, mainly with regard to domestic tasks and partially personal care. The limitations of regarding support for long-term care needs as a social right are also suggested by local variations to be observed, first of all in Italy, but also in Austria and the United Kingdom. On the other hand, payment for care programmes do establish a social right. This is strongest in Austria, where there is just one payment programme with clear eligibility criteria and a legally enforceable right to these benefits. In the United Kingdom, a variety of cash payments with different eligibility criteria exist. In Italy broad local variations are to be observed that do not correspond with differences in health related aspects. Finally, in the Netherlands the personal budget programme is on the one hand strictly limited with respect to the overall budget available, and on the other hand, it puts strict limits on the actual use of the money. Hence, with regard to cash benefits, limits are strongest in the Netherlands.

Extending choice and extending social rights in long-term care has important implications with regard to preserve dignity and to reduce socially excluding effects. Such effects might occur when long-term care systems are designed according to the social assistance idea. This is the case in Italy and Austria where the finance of residential care includes not just financial resources of those in need of care, but also – with substantial room for discretion – that of close family members. In Austria, cash benefits introduced in 1993 are an important relief in this respect. Recent policy initiatives promoting care in the community or establishing standards for long-term care are major attempts to strengthen social inclusion of those in need of care.

It is again the sphere of informal care-giving where attempts to reduce socially excluding effects are only in its infancy, if such attempts exist at all. A number of studies have shown that informal long-term care is not just a physically burdensome and often unrecognised job. Long hours of informal care work as well as care work alongside work in the regular labour market have multiple negative effects on the main care giver. Apart from the effects on the actual or future position in the labour market and in the social protection system, a number of studies have identified negative effects on the carers' health status as well as social integration within family and wider social networks.

With regard to social integration, information on choices and possibilities as well as the ability to decide are most important, for those in need of care as well as care givers. This can be achieved by a mix of policies, including the design of policies and the promotion of interests. Universal programmes, such as the Austrian payment for care programme, are much easier to access and to administer than the range of payment programmes existing in the United Kingdom. With regard to social services, choice requires easy access to a variety of services, by for example establishing a single access point for the whole range of potential services to be used. This is realised most in the Netherlands. The same is true for informal carers' support, which however lacks a much more clear support strategy. Carers associations as existing in the United Kingdom and to a smaller extent in the Netherlands as well as various tools to improve information have a major role of promoting carers interests, by informing carers as well as policy makers.

The objective of social integration with respect to those in need of care is promoted in all the countries under consideration, in particular by extending payment for care programmes and diversifying social services. Whereas steps towards inclusion for people in need of care are taken, this is not the case for informal care givers. Individual burdens are still enormous, in particular in the case of long-lasting severe care needs. As with the economic objectives, informal carers remain in a most precarious situation. Public support is still very much limited and does not prevent people from economic and social exclusion.

In conclusion, the analysis shows that equity choices in long-term care are characterised by an enormous complexity with regard to all the dimensions examined in this study. Investigating to what extent these choices support the achievement of specific equity objectives underlines that the design of long-term care systems does not follow a clear concept of equity objectives. (For a summary see Tables 5.6 and 5.7) A clear countrywide approach just exists in the Netherlands. In Austria and even more so in Italy, apart from cash benefits, territorial variations in service supply are probably the main characteristic in their long-term care system, though in the 1990s Austria has already undertaken major steps to reduce these inequalities by introducing a universal payment for care programme and co-ordinating the development of social services across the country. The United Kingdom is a mixture of all the 'models', combining a broad range of social services including novel approaches in managing these services as well as cash programmes and establishing clear public responsibilities alongside strong private responsibilities.

On a very general level, two issues occur from the choices made in the four countries: Public support is strongest in the Netherlands, followed by the United Kingdom and Austria. These two countries take different places in the hierarchy looking at specific aspects of the long-term care system. Given the overall involvement of the public sector in long-term care measured in terms of spending they are rather close (OECD 1999). Lowest in the ranking in terms of public support and intervention is Italy.

With regard to ranking, choices made are in line with what one might expect from looking at existing welfare state classifications. (see chapter 4.2) On the other hand, the design of long-term care policies differs quite considerably from that in other social policy fields. In health care, for example, the design is very much emphasising the objective of horizontal equality promoting equal access according to need on a rather high level. This is true for all European Countries. A high level of support in terms of replacement ratios as well as coverage is also reached in pension systems. In long-term care, there obviously is no such general policy approach to be observed. Although long-term care is partly seen as public responsibility, and in many countries increasingly so, this responsibility is at the same time clearly limited. To some extent recent policy reforms are aimed at a clarification of rights and responsibilities in long-term care, by designing universal payment for care programmes, standardising needs assessment procedures or by clarifying access to specific services. In this respect, there even is some convergence between the four countries. At the same time, considerable room remains for discretionary decisions and implicit principles in allocation.

Table 5.6 Promoting equity objectives with regard to care receivers

Equity objectives	Austria	Italy	Netherlands	United Kingdom
Guaranteeing minimum standards	yes (private obligations extended to family)	yes (private obligations extended to family)	equity choices going beyond this objective	yes (no extended family obligations)
Supporting living standards	limited, but improved through cash benefits	limited, enormous local variations	yes, but increasingly limited with regard to personal care and domestic help	yes, but increasingly limited with regard to stricter needs-assessment
Reducing horizontal inequality	limited, but improved through cash benefits	limited, enormous local variations	yes, but increasingly limited with regard to personal care and domestic help	yes, but increasingly limited with regard to stricter needs-assessment
Reducing vertical inequality	very limited	very limited	very limited	very limited
Enhancing personal autonomy	improving, limitations with regard to services and co-payments	improving, limitations with regard to services, co-payments and local variations	yes, but increasing limitations with personal care and domestic help	yes, but actual choice increasingly depends on private resources
Equalising social rights and responsibilities	yes with regard to cash benefits, limited with regard to services	limited with regard to cash payments and services	yes	yes, but increasing variations with decentralisation

Table 5.7 Promoting equity objectives with regard to informal care givers

Equity objectives	Austria	Italy	Netherlands	United Kingdom
Guaranteeing minimum standards	yes, as part of other minimum standard schemes	yes, as part of other minimum standard schemes	yes, as part of other minimum standard schemes	yes, including cash benefits to care givers
Supporting living standards	no specific policy measures, importance of intra-family distributions			
	limited indirect effects from cash benefits and access to services	limited indirect effects from cash benefits and access to services	indirect support from a broad range of services	limited indirect effects from cash benefits and access to services
Reducing horizontal inequality	no specific policy measures, importance of intra-family distributions			
	limited indirect effects from cash benefits and access to services	limited indirect effects from cash benefits and access to services	indirect support from a broad range of services	limited indirect effects from cash benefits and access to services
Reducing vertical inequality	very limited	very limited	very limited	very limited
Enhancing personal autonomy	very limited specific measures (just short term leaves, very little support regarding coverage in social protection schemes)			
	otherwise, indirect effects according to the availability of and access to services and benefits			
Equalising social rights and responsibilities	very limited specific social rights with regard to the role as informal care giver			
	obligation of maintenance for close family members, considerable room for discretionary measures	obligation of maintenance for close family members, considerable room for discretionary measures	no legal obligation for family members	no legal obligation, but family resources are increasingly recognised in the assessment of care needs

6 Conclusions

In this concluding chapter the main issues of the study will be revisited and discussed in a broader welfare state perspective. In the first part it looks at welfare state objectives and choices, arguing that the approach followed in this study is an important addition to existing strands in equity research. It recognises the complexity of choices and offers an innovative framework going beyond traditional concepts. In the second part, a brief summary and outlook is given with regard to similarities, differences and trends in equity choices and long-term care policies.

What choices, what equity?

Objectives of welfare and the welfare state conflict and people disagree upon the importance of different objectives. Disagreement and dispute arise with regard to definition, compatibility, or ranking of major objectives such as efficiency, freedom, and equity. Disagreements arise from differences in value systems, from beliefs and assessments with regard to the adequacy of objectives, specific measures as means to support specific objectives or the implications of respective measures. Statements regarding equity as a welfare state objective are attractive in policy making as well as in researching welfare issues. Even when cost-containment and efficiency-improving approaches come to the forefront in welfare state policies, equity is a major argument for promoting reforms. Statements explicitly defining equity as a major concern in long-term care policies are, however, rare. But debates on the finance of long-term care or on the division of public and private responsibilities clearly point at the importance of equity issues in long-term care.

This book has been developing 'equity choices' as an analytic framework to systematically analyse choices reflecting different equity interpretations in the welfare state. In the conclusion, three issues regarding choices and equity in welfare state research will be revisited: the role of the analytic framework in equity research, equity choices as an extension of existing analytic concepts in comparative welfare state research, and further applications of the framework.

'Equity choices' as an addition to equity research: Without further clarification equity remains a rather elusive issue. The gap between rhetoric

and practice and between ideal equity concepts and societal outcome is enormous. There are various approaches to bring substance to the concept of equity, mostly in normative and empirical equity research. The approach of these strands in equity research is either prescriptive (how equity ought to be defined), the major focus is on testing specific interpretations of equity, or on studying what the people think equity is. Given the focus of these strands and the complexity of equity, their potential to actually bridge the above mentioned gap is limited. Inequalities observed in empirical equity research provide interesting information on the structure of inequalities. But there often is no or very little discussion on the relevance of the underlying equity interpretation, nor are the results of testing specific interpretations – given the design of the respective policy field – much of a surprise.

As a consequence, this study has attempted to bring the design of equity interpretations to the core of the approach. Three key elements of such interpretations have been identified: what is to be allocated, among whom, and according to which principles. The what question refers to cash benefits or in-kind services, cash or in-kind burdens, and/or the regulation of these resources and burdens. Behind these more visible resources, policies are aimed at access, use, choice, and outcome. The focal subjects of allocation are individuals, (potential) care receivers and (potential) care givers, as well as families, households, companies or local public bodies as intermediate focal subjects. Finally, need-related variables, time-related variables, economic variables or status variables are applied as single or mixed principles and determine, alongside implicit principles, the actual allocation of resources and burdens. The conceptual and empirical analysis has shown that respective choices by welfare states are a complex combination of various resources and burdens to be shared, different units among whom these goods are shared and principles that are often used as mixed principles in the actual allocation leaving also room for additional implicit principles.

This approach allows equity to be studied in the welfare state as it is translated into welfare state practice. It does not start from any predefined equity interpretation, but uses the design of the provision and the finance of welfare as reflections of underlying welfare state objectives. As Miller (1992) has used the expression 'What the people think' as a description of empirical equity research, the concept of 'equity choices' in the context of welfare state research could be described as 'What welfare states do'.

'Equity choices' as an extension of analytic concepts: Debating and studying the design of welfare systems tends to be focused on basic principles or concepts. Universality vs. selectivity, social rights vs.

insurance vs. assistance, cash benefits vs. in kind benefits, etc. are important examples for such principles. These principles are guiding the design of welfare policies. They have been used as indicators to describe and to cluster welfare state families. And they reflect diverse ideas about the allocation of resources and burdens and contain different interpretations regarding equity and equity objectives. Their capacity to assess the actual design of allocations and respective equity implications has, however, its limitations and does not reflect the broad range of details in welfare state design, as will be shown by some examples.

The distinction between liberal, corporatist and universal welfare states or between social assistance, social insurance, and universal social protection models is at the core of comparative welfare state research. The distinction has considerable potential to inform about various welfare state families, what to be expected from the design of the respective welfare state policies, or the implications regarding the distribution of resources and burdens. With regard to long-term care, the countries studied here follow these models in terms of the ranking in the overall extent of public intervention. But – and this has also been shown earlier (e.g. Alber 1995, Anttonen, Sipilä 1996) – major long-term care features are either neglected in the analyses or the respective long-term care systems deviate from what is suggested by these model types. Finance is not primarily based on social insurance contributions in any of the four countries, rather on taxes. Social assistance plays a rather strong role, whereas existing universal benefits are very limited. And, long-term care is characterised by a considerable amount of informal care-giving. It is the major burden in financing long-term care in all countries, which however is almost neglected with regard to opportunity costs arising to those providing informal care-giving, gender inequalities in the distribution of informal care-giving, or the implications with regard to inclusion in the labour market and social protection schemes.

The same is true for the universality – selectivity dichotomy. Long-term care policies are not just about selectivity or universality, but about what type of selectivity. In long-term care, selectivity is based on a mix of different criteria, including means-testing, out-of-pocket payments, huge variations in the definition of need, waiting lists, and a broad range of implicit criteria. Criteria also varying within single countries and with regard to different forms of providing long-term care, further expand the mix of allocation principles used in practice. Starting from the concepts of universality and selectivity or the concepts of social assistance, social insurance and universal social protection in comparative welfare state research is a helpful tool for clustering welfare states. But the broad range of potential choices embedded in any of these concepts tends to remain invisible.

Another example is the distinction made between regulation, cash benefits and in-kind support as types of welfare state intervention. Regarding long-term care in Europe, a clear distinction can be made between the northern European countries offering high levels of in-kind support but limited cash benefits, to the United Kingdom with a combination of both, and most other European countries with a partly fragmented residential and domiciliary care sector and evolving payment for care programmes. Cash and in-kind emphasise different aspects with regard to equity. From the ideal type perspective, cash payments tend to emphasise freedom of choice creating an opportunity to have access to and to use specific services, whereas in-kind benefits are aimed at the provision of specific qualities. But again, in practice programmes differ widely with regard to the actual design and underlying equity interpretations. For example, a highly regulated personal budget system in the Netherlands restricts freedom of choice to specific choice sets, which on the other hand guarantees specific use of these payments. Cash payments in Austria and in Italy are a contribution to cover extra-costs of care without defining how payments have to be used. In terms of equity implications, the cash benefit programme in the Netherlands comes much closer to in-kind benefits than the cash benefit programmes in Austria and in Italy.

Institutional arrangements are another prominent approach in comparative welfare state research. Long-term care is a prime example for the welfare mix, combining actors in the public sector, in the non-profit and – to a much smaller extent – the for-profit sector as well as actors in the informal sphere including families, households and other informal networks. Any of these institutional settings is characterised by specific principles of co-ordination, allocation and eligibility and, hence, has its potential and problems. (see chapter 3.3) Important potential equity implications are rooted in the specific rules of the four settings. But actual outcomes might differ quite widely depending on the broad range of choices covered by the equity choices approach. For example, payments for care made to care receivers or informal care givers will affect the relationship between various actors, decisions with regard to providing and financing care-giving, and intra-family distributions. Another example is the allocation of decision-making power. Shifting global budgets and decision-making power to local authorities produces quite distinct outcomes compared to systems characterised by well-defined countrywide standards. Not just in long-term care, there is a tendency towards decentralisation, contracting out, and managerialism in the public sector.

Primarily aimed at increasing efficiency and improving targeting, it creates new explicit and implicit criteria for allocating resources and burdens and, hence, equity implications.

Focusing welfare state analysis on choices regarding objects, subjects and principles of allocation goes beyond basic principles, as briefly shown by the examples above. It offers an opportunity to comparatively study welfare state responses to specific problems in social policy covering the objects of allocation, that is the whole range of resources and burdens that might be allocated, the subjects of allocation, that is final and intermediate units allocation might be aimed at, as well as the principles of allocation, that is the criteria to decide upon the respective shares. Such an approach recognises the complexity of such choices and the richness of welfare state design. At the same time it offers an accurate framework for systematically investigating equity.

Further applications of the framework: In this book the framework has been used to study equity choices in long-term care in a cross-country perspective and to contrast actual choices with equity objectives. Moreover, the analytic concept provides a starting point for a wide range of further research questions. The framework might be used for analysing equity interpretations in other social policy fields, or in comparing different areas of welfare state intervention. It allows approaching equity in comparative perspective as well as in a single country perspective or even smaller scale units. Equity choices offer an accurate tool for equity research focusing on specific actors (not just the welfare state) designing or making equity choices as well as equity research focusing on those affected by such choices. Equity choices could be the starting point for the analysis of causal factors for specific choices or the consequences of choices on welfare state objectives other than equity. Hence, equity choices can help to connect normative ideas about equity and the actual distribution of resources and burdens.

What future for long-term care policies?

Because of demographic and socio-economic changes and challenges, cost-containment and efficiency-improving approaches have recently been dominating welfare state policies. Many reforms are very much driven by these concerns, in long-term care (Glendinning, Schunk, McLaughlin 1997) as in other areas of social policy. Related issues are measures to reduce the length of stay in hospitals, they include approaches to reduce or to stabilise the number of beds in residential care settings, to shift care-giving responsibilities from residential care settings to the community, to concentrate public support on those with more extended care-needs, the search for private solutions in financing and providing care, etc. But this did not necessarily come along with a reduction in overall public long-term care spending. Apart from the Nordic countries, the Netherlands and to a smaller extent the United Kingdom, long-term care systems were and partly still are rather fragmented, with social services or residential care settings completely lacking or varying across countries and across regions, cash benefits being rather limited, and social assistance being a major principle in the design of benefits.

Alongside cost-containment concerns, and partly as a consequence, objectives such as choice, quality and autonomy have received increasing recognition in recent policy debates. In this respect, a diversification in long-term care systems offering opportunities between the traditional approach of residential or domiciliary care as well as measures to integrate the various services, can be observed. But, at the same time, access to specific services is reduced by stricter needs assessment including the availability of family care, which in turn reduces room for individual choice given the costs of care. Regarding personal autonomy, those in need of care have received some recognition through the improvement and diversification of services just mentioned as well as payment for care programmes. Informal care givers have been addressed only more recently, with the actual support being still very small regarding the enormous burdens and opportunity costs connected with long-term care.

European countries are far from having an agreement about general equity objectives in long-term care (see chapter 5.3). Current approaches in the actual design of the respective systems differ widely (see chapters 5.1 and 5.2). Summarising recent policy developments as revealed in European long-term care policies, the following trends might be expected: It is regarded as public responsibility to cover or at least to considerably contribute to nursing care and the needs of the most severely disabled people, whereas personal care and, even more so, domestic tasks are seen as shared or private responsibility. For medical and nursing related care, policies promote the objective of horizontal equality and that of supporting living standards. For personal care and domestic tasks there is some financial support, but restricted either by means-testing or contributions covering just part of the costs and, hence, promoting the objective of guaranteeing a minimum standard rather than supporting living standards and horizontal equality. Such an approach of clarifying public and private responsibilities might, in the medium run, reduce some inequalities, including territorial inequalities as well as the range of implicit principles producing such inequalities. Approaches strengthening decentralised decision-making may, however, have an opposite effect if room for discretionary decisions and standards for these decisions are rather vague.

With regard to policies aimed at those offering informal long-term care no such trends can be observed. There is a huge gap between rhetoric and practice. The recognition of informal long-term care in public policies is still in its infancy. Aspects of economic and social integration of informal care givers have been ignored in countries characterised by high levels of support and in countries characterised by low levels of public provision, even if for very different reasons. The recognition of emotional relationships in caring and specific burdens rooted in here is low. There are some attempts to recognise informal long-term care-giving through payment for care programmes and the inclusion in parts of the social protection system. At the same time, however, the role of informal care givers might become even more precarious when welfare benefits are increasingly attached to participation in formal employment and responsibilities for personal care and domestic tasks are – for reasons of financial constraints – shifted back to the private sphere. As a consequence, this will often increase informal obligations and opportunity costs. This aspect mainly affects women given the actual intra-family distribution of these obligations. Approaches to reduce inequalities between men and women in the distribution of these obligations do not exist.

This study has been driven by an interest in two themes: Equity, and how it looks like in translating it into 'real world', and long-term care, and how welfare states intervene in the provision and in the finance of long-term care. Long-term care – more than any other social policy field characterised by a broad diversity of policies and institutions, tensions and dependencies between formal and informal activities, paid and unpaid work, professionals and non-professionals – offers a unique opportunity to study these issues. Despite the differences in the status quo of designing long-term care systems and differences in the social and economic background, the study also shows some common trends towards a clarification of public and private responsibilities in long-term care. With regard to informal care givers, similarities stand for implicit effects and very little specific social policy support leaving informal carers in a burdensome, unstable and dependent situation. Here, the study points at a huge deficit in social policy and suggests major efforts to improve the most precarious situation of informal carers offering long hours of care. On a more general level, it suggests to strengthen discourse on the plurality of objectives in welfare state policies and on objects, subjects and principles of allocating resources and burdens.

Glossary

domestic help	helping in the household with e.g. cleaning, washing, cooking, shopping, preparing food, etc.
domiciliary care	care provided in the home of the person in need of care (= home care); including nursing care, personal care and domestic help
home care	care provided in the home of the person in need of care (= domiciliary care); including nursing care, personal care and domestic help
home help	domestic help provided in the home of the person in need of care (this also might include personal care)
home nursing	specialised nursing care provided in the home of the person in need of care (this also might include personal care)
informal care giver	anyone engaged in looking after a spouse, relative, neighbour or friend who is ill or disabled and needs help or support in nursing, personal or domestic tasks, without being on a regular contract for fulfilling these tasks
institutional care	residence and care provided in an institution to individuals in need of care, in particular in nursing homes and residential homes (= residential care)
long-term care	any care provided consistently over an extended period of time, with no predetermined finishing date, to a person with a long-standing limiting condition or who is at risk of neglect or injury (definition following Kalisch, Aman, Buchele 1998)

long-term care dependency ratio	number of people in need of long-term care as a proportion of those of working age; usually defined as those in need of long-term care as a percentage of those aged 15 to 65 years of age
nursing care	nursing activities related to illnesses and medical problems; e.g. dressing wounds, administering injections, etc.
nursing home	institutional (residential) care setting providing accommodation, meals, personal care and nursing care
old-age dependency ratio	number of elderly people who are not of working age as a proportion of those of working age; usually defined as those aged aged 65 and over as a percentage of those aged 15 to 65 years of age
payments for care	cash payments for care given either to care receivers or to informal care givers
personal care	help to assist people with their activities of daily living related to the own body; e.g. eating, personal hygiene, dressing, etc.
residential care	residence and care provided in an institution to individuals in need of care, in particular in nursing homes and residential homes (= institutional care)
residential home	institutional (residential) care setting providing accommodation, meals and to some extent personal care
respite care	professional care provided to offer relief and breaks from care-giving tasks to informal care-givers
total dependency ratio	number of people who are not of working age as a proportion of those of working age; usually defined as those aged under 15 years and those aged 65 and over as a percentage of those aged 15 to 65 years of age

Bibliography

Alber, J. (1995): A Framework for the Comparative Study of Social Services, in: Journal of European Social Policy, Vol. 5, No. 2, 131-149

Aldridge, J., Becker, S. (1996): Caught in the Caring Trap. The Health of Children who Care, in: Bywaters, P., McLeod, E. (Eds.): Working for Equality in Health, London: Routledge

Allen, I., Perkins, E. (Eds.) (1995): The Future of Family Care for Older People, London: HMSO

Amaradio, L. (1998): Financing Long-Term Care for Elderly Persons: What are the Options?, in: Journal of Health Care Financing, Vol. 25, No. 2, 75-84

Anttonen, A., Sipilä, J. (1996): European Social Care Services: Is it Possible to Identify Models?, in: Journal of European Social Policy, Vol. 6, No. 2, 87-100

Arber, S., Ginn, J. (1991): Gender and Later Life: A Sociological Analysis of Resources and Constraints, London: Sage

Arber, S., Ginn, J. (1995): Gender Differences in the Relationship between Paid Employment and Informal Care, in: Work, Employment & Society, Vol. 9, No. 3, 445-471

Arneson, R. (1989): Equality and Equality of Opportunity for Welfare, in: Philosophical Studies, Vol. 56, No. 1, 77-93

Atkinson, A.B., Stiglitz, J.E. (1980): Lectures on Public Economics, London: McGraw Hill

Badelt, C. (1998): Zwischen Marktversagen und Staatsversagen? Nonprofit Organisationen aus sozioökonomischer Sicht, in: Badelt, C. (Ed.): Handbuch der Nonprofit Organisation. Strukturen und Entwicklungstrends. 2nd Edition, Stuttgart: Schaeffer-Poeschel

Badelt, C. (1999): The Role of NPOs in Policies to Combat Social Exclusion, Social Protection Discussion Paper No. 9912, Washington: World Bank

Badelt, C., Holzmann-Jenkins, A., Matul, C., Österle, A. (1997): Analyse der Auswirkungen des Pflegevorsorgesystems, Wien: BMAGS

Badelt, C., Holzmann, A., Matul, C., Österle, A. (1996): Kosten der Pflegesicherung. Strukturen und Entwicklungstrends der Altenbetreuung. 2nd Edition, Wien: Böhlau Verlag

Badelt, C., Leichsenring, K. (2000): Versorgung, Betreuung, Pflege, in: Ältere Menschen – Neue Perspektiven. Seniorenbericht 2000: Zur Lebenssituation älterer Menschen in Österreich, Wien: Bundesministerium für soziale Sicherheit und Generationen

Badelt, C., Österle, A. (2001a): Grundzüge der Sozialpolitik. Allgemeiner Teil: Sozialökonomische Grundlagen. 2nd Edition, Wien: Manz

Badelt, C., Österle, A. (2001b): Grundzüge der Sozialpolitik. Spezieller Teil: Sozialpolitik in Österreich. 2nd Edition, Wien: Manz

Baldock, J. (1993): Home and Community-Based Services for the Elderly in the United Kingdom, in: Lesemann, Martin (1993)

Baldock, J. (1997): Social Care in Old Age: More than a Funding Problem, in: Social Policy & Administration, Vol. 31, No. 1, 73-89

Baldock, J., Ely, P. (1996): Social Care for Elderly People in Europe. The Central Problem of Home Care, in: Munday, P., Ely, P. (Eds.): Social Care in Europe, London: Prentice Hall

Baldock, J., Ungerson, C. (1991): 'What d'ya want if you don' want money?'. A Feminist Critique of 'Paid Volunteering', in: Maclean, M., Groves, D. (Eds.): Women's Issues in Social Policy, London: Routledge

Barr, N. (1998): The Economics of the Welfare State. 3rd Edition, Oxford: Oxford University Press

Barry, B. (1989): Theories of Justice, Berkeley: University of California Press

Barta, H., Ganner, M. (Eds.) (1998): Alter, Recht und Gesellschaft. Rechtliche Rahmenbedingungen der Alten- und Pflegebetreuung, Wien: WUV-Universitätsverlag

Bebbington, A.C., Davies, B. (1983): Equity and Efficiency in the Allocation of the Personal Social Services, in: Journal of Social Policy, Vol. 12, No. 3, 309-330

Bell, J. (1992): Justice and the Law, in: Scherer (1992)

Bell, J., Schokkaert, E. (1992): Interdisciplinary Theory and Research on Justice, in: Scherer (1992)

Belletti, F., Keen, H. (1999): Social Protection for Dependency in Old Age in Italy. National Report Series for the Social Protection for Dependency in Old Age in the 15 EU Member States and Norway Project, Leuven: HIVA

Beltrametti, L. (1998): L'assistenza ai non autosufficienti: Alcuni elementi per il dibattito, in: Politica Economica, Vol. XIV, No. 1, 155-185

Berthold, N. (1988): Marktversagen, staatliche Intervention und Organisationsformen sozialer Sicherung, in: Rolf, G., Spahn, P.B., Wagner, G. (Eds.): Sozialvertrag und Soziale Sicherung. Zur ökonomischen Theorie staatlicher Versicherungs- und Umverteilungssysteme, Frankfurt: Campus

Bettio, F., Prechal, S. (1998): Care in Europe. Joint Report of the 'Gender and Employment' and the 'Gender and Law' Groups of Experts, Brussels: European Commission

Binstock, R.H. (1998): The Financing and Organisation of Long-Term Care, in: Walker, Bradley, Wetle (1998)

Binstock, R.H., Post, S. (Eds.) (1991): Too Old for Health Care? Controversies in Medicine, Law, Economics and Ethics, Baltimore: Johns Hopkins University Press

Blankart, C.B. (1991): Öffentliche Finanzen in der Demokratie: Einführung in die Finanzwissenschaft, München: Vahlen

BMAGS (Ed.) (1999a): Bericht des Arbeitskreises für Pflegevorsorge 1998, Wien: Bundesministerium für Arbeit, Gesundheit und Soziales

BMAGS (Ed.) (1999b): Dienste und Einrichtungen für pflegebedürftige Menschen in Österreich. Übersicht über die Bedarfs- und Entwicklungspläne der Länder, Wien: Bundesministerium für Arbeit, Gesundheit und Soziales

BMSG (Ed.) (2000): Bericht des Arbeitskreises für Pflegevorsorge 1999, Wien: Bundesministerium für soziale Sicherheit und Generationen

Bond, J., Buck, D. (1999): Social Protection for Dependency in Old Age in the United Kingdom. National Report Series for the Social Protection for Dependency in Old Age in the 15 EU Member States and Norway Project, Leuven: HIVA

Bonoli, G. (1997): Classifying Welfare States: A Two Dimensional Approach, in: Journal of Social Policy, Vol. 26, No. 3, 351-372

Bradley, E.H. (1998): Self-interested Behaviour and Social Welfare: Perspectives from Economic Theory, in: Walker, Bradley, Wetle (1998)

Bradshaw, J. (1972): A Taxonomy of Social Need, in: McLachlan, G. (Ed.): Problems and Progress in Medical Care: Essays on Current Research. 7th Series, London: Oxford University Press

Brodsky, J., Habib, J., Mizrahi, I. (2000): Long-Term Care Laws in Five Developed Countries. A Review, Geneva: World Health Organization

Byrne, D. (1999): Social Exclusion, Buckingham: Open University Press

Calabresi, G., Bobbit, P. (1978): Tragic Choices, New York: Norton

Cambois, E., Robine, J.-M. (1996): An International Comparison of Trends in Disability Free Life Expectancy, in: Eisen, Sloan (1996)

Carmichael, F., Charles, S. (1998): The Labour Market Costs of Community Care, in: Journal of Health Economics, Vol. 17, No. 6, 747-765

Castles, F. (Ed.) (1993): Families of Nations: Patterns of Public Policies in Western Democracies, Aldershot: Dartmouth

Clarke, L. (1995): Family Care and Changing Family Structure: Bad News for the Elderly, in: Allen, Perkins (1995)

Clasen, J. (Ed.) (1999): Comparative Social Policy. Concepts, Theories and Methods, Oxford: Blackwell

Clement, G. (1998): Care, Autonomy, and Justice. Feminism and the Ethic of Care, Oxford: Westview Press

Cohen, G. (1989): On the Currency of Egalitarian Justice, in: Ethics, Vol. 99, 906-944

Coolen, J., Weekers, S. (1998): Long-Term Care in The Netherlands: Public Funding and Private Provision within a Universalistic Welfare State, in: Glendinning (1998a)

Coughlin, T.A., McBride, T.D., Perozek, M., Liu, K. (1992): Home Care for the Disabled Elderly: Predictors and Expected Costs, in: Health Services Research, Vol. 27, No. 4, 453-479

Cullis, J., Jones, P. (1998): Public Finance and Public Choice. 2nd Edition, Oxford: Oxford University Press

Culyer, A.J. (1980): The Political Economy of Social Policy, Oxford: Martin Robertson

Daly, M. (1994): Comparing Welfare States: Towards a Gender Friendly Approach, in: Sainsbury, D. (Ed.): Gendering Welfare States, London: Sage

Daly, M. (2000): The Gender Division of Welfare, Cambridge: Cambridge University Press

Daniels, N. (1985): Just Health Care, Cambridge: Cambridge University Press

Daniels, N. (1988): Am I My Parents Keeper?, New York: Oxford University Press

Davies, B. (1987): Equity and Efficiency in Community Care: Supply and Financing in an Age of Fiscal Austerity, in: Ageing and Society, Vol. 7, 161-174

Davies, B. (1988): Financing Long-Term Social Care: Challenges for the Nineties, in: Social Policy and Administration, Vol. 22, No. 2, 97-114

Davies, B., Fernández, J., Saunders, R. (1999): Community Care in England and France. Reforms and the Improvement of Equity and Efficiency, Aldershot: Ashgate

Davies, B., Fernández, J., Nomer, B. (2000): Equity and Efficiency in Policy in Community Care. Needs, Service Productivities, Efficiencies and their Implications, Aldershot: Ashgate

Davies, B.P., Knapp, M. (1981): Old People's Homes and the Production of Welfare, London: Routledge & Kegan Paul

Davis, K., Rowland, D. (1986): Medicare Policies: New Directions for Health and Long-Term Care, Baltimore: Johns Hopkins University Press

Department of Health (1998): Independent Inquiry into Inequalities in Health. Report, London: Stationary Office

Ditch, J., Barnes, H., Bradshaw, J., Kilkey, M. (1998): A Synthesis of National Family Policies 1996. European Observatory on National Family Policies, Luxembourg: European Commission

Dobson, A. (1998): Justice and the Environment. Conceptions of Environmental Sustainability and Dimensions of Social Justice, Oxford: Oxford University Press

Doty, P. (1988): Long-Term Care in International Perspective, in: Health Care Financing Review, Annual Supplement, 145-155

Doty, P., Jackson, M.E., Crown, W. (1998): The Impact of Female Caregivers' Employment Status on Patterns of Formal and Informal Eldercare, in: The Gerontologist, Vol. 38, No. 3, 331-341

Doyal, L., Gough, I. (1991): A Theory of Human Need, London: Macmillan

Dworkin, R. (1981a): What is Equality? Part I: Equality of Welfare, in: Philosophy and Public Affairs, Vol. 10, No. 3, 185-247

Dworkin, R. (1981b): What is Equality? Part I: Equality of Resources, in: Philosophy and Public Affairs, Vol. 10, No. 4, 283-345

Edvartsen, T.O. (1996): Possibilities and Problems in a Cross-Country Comparative Analysis of Long-Term Care Systems, in: Eisen, Sloan (1996)

Eger, T., Weise, P. (1998): Gutscheine und Zertifikate, in: Tietzel (1998)

Eisen, R. (1992): Alternative Sicherungsmöglichkeiten bei Pflegebedürftigkeit, in: Sozialer Fortschritt, Vol. 41, No. 10, 236-241

Eisen, R., Mager, H.-C. (Eds.) (2000): Pflegebedürftigkeit und Pflegesicherung in ausgewählten Ländern, Opladen: Leske und Budrich

Eisen, R., Sloan, F.A. (Eds.) (1996): Long-Term Care: Economic Issues and Policy Solutions, Dordrecht: Kluwer

Eliasson Lappalainen, R., Nilsson Motevasel, I. (1997): Ethics of Care and Social Policy, in: Scandinavian Journal of Social Welfare, Vol. 6, No. 2, 189-196

Ellis, K., Davis, A., Rummery, K. (1999): Needs Assessment, Street-Level Bureaucracy and the New Community Care, in: Social Policy & Administration, Vol. 33, No. 3, 262-280

Elster, J. (1992): Local Justice. How Institutions Allocate Scarce Goods and Necessary Burdens, New York: Russel Sage Foundation

Engelstad, F. (Ed.) (1994): Layoffs and Local Justice, Oslo: Institute for Social Research

Esping-Anderson, G. (1990): The Three Worlds of Welfare Capitalism, Cambridge: Polity Press

Esping-Andersen, G. (Ed.) (1996): Welfare States in Transition. National Adaptations in Global Economies, London: Sage

Ettner, S.L. (1996): The Opportunity Cost of Elder Care, in: The Journal of Human Resources, Vol. 31, No. 1, 189-205

European Commission (1998): Social Protection in Europe 1997, Luxembourg: Office for Official Publications of the European Communities

Eurostat (Ed.) (1997): Demographic Statistics 1997, Luxembourg: Office for Official Publications of the European Communities

Evandrou, M., Falkingham, J., Le Grand, J., Winter, D. (1992): Equity in Health and Social Care, in: Journal of Social Policy, Vol. 21, No. 4, 489-523

Evers, A. (1994): Payments for Care: A Small but Significant Part of a Wider Debate, in: Evers, Pijl, Ungerson (1994)

Evers, A., Leichsenring, K., Pruckner, B. (1994): Payments for Care. The Case of Austria, in: Evers, Pijl, Ungerson (1994)

Evers, A., Olk, T. (1996): Wohlfahrtspluralismus – Analytische und normativ-politische Dimensionen eines Leitbegriffs, in: Evers, A., Olk, T. (Eds.): Wohlfahrtspluralismus. Vom Wohlfahrtsstaat zur Wohlfahrtsgesellschaft, Opladen: Westdeutscher Verlag

Evers, A., Pijl, M., Ungerson, C. (Eds.) (1994): Payments for Care: A Comparative Overview, Aldershot: Avebury

Evers, A., Svetlik, I. (Eds.) (1993): Balancing Pluralism. New Welfare Mixes in Care for the Elderly, Aldershot: Avebury

Facchini, C., Scortegagna, R. (1993): Home Care Services for the Elderly in Italy, in: Lesemann, Martin (1993)

Felder, S., Zweifel, P. (1998): Provision and Financing of Long-Term Care for the Elderly: The Role of Government, in: Marmor, T.R., De Jong, P.R. (Eds.): Ageing, Social Security and Affordability, Aldershot: Ashgate

Ferrera, M. (1993): Modelli di solidarietà. Politica e riforme sociali nelle democrazie, Bologna: Il Mulino

Ferrera, M. (1996): The 'Southern Model' of Welfare in Social Europe, in: Journal of European Social Policy, Vol. 6, No. 1, 17-37

Finch, J. (1989): Family Obligations and Social Change, Cambridge: Polity Press

Finch, J., Mason, J. (1993): Negotiating Family Responsibilities, London: Tavistock

Fisher, M. (1994): Man-Made Care: Community Care and Older Male Carers, in: British Journal of Social Work, Vol. 24, 59-80

Fleurbaey, M. (1995): Equal Opportunity or Equal Social Outcome, in: Economics and Philosophy, Vol. 11, 25-55

Folland, S., Goodman, A.C., Stano, M. (1997): The Economics of Health and Health Care, Upper Saddle River: Prentice Hall

Fox, J. (Ed.) (1989): Inequalities in European Countries, Aldershot: Gower

Fries, J.F. (1980): Aging, Natural Death, and the Compression of Morbidity, in: New England Journal of Medicine, No. 303, 130-135

Fuchs, V.R. (1974): Who Shall Live?, New York: Basic Books

Garber, A.M. (1996): To Comfort Always: The Prospects of Expanded Social Responsibility for Long-Term Care, in: Fuchs, V.R. (Ed.): Individual and Social Responsibility, Chicago: University of Chicago Press

George, V. (1996): The Demand for Welfare, in: George, Vic, Taylor-Gooby, Peter (Eds.): European Welfare Policy. Squaring the Welfare Circle, London: Macmillan

Giarchi, G.G. (1996): Caring for Older Europeans, Comparative Studies in 29 Countries, Aldershot: Ashgate

Gibson, D. (1998): Aged Care. Old Policies, New Problems, Cambridge: Cambridge University Press

Gilbert, N., Specht, H., Terrell, P. (1993): Dimensions of Social Welfare Policy. 3rd Edition, Englewood Cliffs: Prentice Hall

Gillon, R. (1986): Philosophical Medical Ethics, Chichester: John Wiley

Glendinning, C. (1992): Employment and 'Community Care'. Policies for the 1990s, in: Work, Employment and Society, Vol. 6, No. 1, 103-111

Glendinning, C. (Ed.) (1998a): Rights and Realities. Comparing New Developments in Long-Term Care for Older People, Bristol: Polity Press

Glendinning, C. (1998b): Health and Social Care Services for Frail Older People in the UK: Changing Responsibilities and New Developments, in: Glendinning (1998a)

Glendinning, C., McLaughlin, E. (1993): Paying for Care: Lessons from Europe, London: HMSO

Glendinning, C., Schunk, M., McLaughlin, E. (1997): Paying for Long-Term Domiciliary Care: A Comparative Perspective, in: Ageing and Society, Vol. 17, No. 2, 123-140

Glennerster, H. (1997): Paying for Welfare. Towards 2000. 3rd Edition, London: Prentice Hall

Göke, M., Hartwig, K.-H. (1998): Schwarzmärkte, in: Tietzel (1998)

Goldberg, E.M., Barnes, J., Corcoran, K., Davies, B., Davies, M., Fruin, D., Hardwood, P., Plank, D., Timms, N. (1980): Directions for Research in Social Work and the Social Services, in: British Journal of Social Work, Vol. 10, 207-217

Goodin, R.E., Headey, B., Muffels, R., Dirven, H.-J. (1999): The Real Worlds of Welfare Capitalism, Cambridge: Cambridge University Press

Gori, C. (2000): Solidarity in Italy's Policies Towards the Frail Elderly: A Value at Stake, in: International Journal of Social Welfare, Vol. 9, No. 4, 261-269

Gori, C. (2001): Des situations contrastées au plan territorial: Le cas italien, in: Martin (2001)

Gough, I. (1993): Economic Institutions and Human Well-Being, in: Drover, G., Kerans, P. (Eds.): New Approaches to Welfare Theory, Aldershot: Edward Elgar

Grossman, M. (1972): On the Concept of Health Capital and the Demand for Health, in: Journal of Political Economy, Vol. 80, 223-255

Grundy, E. (1995): Demographic Influences on the Future of Family Care, in: Allen, Perkins (1995)

Hantrais, L. (1994): Family Policy in Europe, in: Page, R., Baldock, J. (Eds.): Social Policy Review, No. 6, Canterbury: SPA

Hantrais, L., Mangen, S. (Eds.) (1996): Cross-National Research Methods in the Social Sciences, London: Pinter

Hauser, R. (1991): Probleme der vergleichenden Analyse von Systemen sozialer Sicherung – Drei Beispiele aus dem Bereich der Alterssicherung, in: Thiemeyer, Theo (Ed.): Theoretische Grundlagen der Sozialpolitik II, Berlin: Duncker&Humblot

Heitzmann, K. (1999): Transitions to Adulthood, Lone Parenthood, Sickness or Disability and Retirement: Empirical Analysis of the ECHP for Austria. Working Paper for the T.S.E.R. Project 'Family Structure, Labour Market Participation and the Dynamics of Social Exclusion', Wien: Wirtschaftsuniversität

Hennessy, P. (1997): Die Zunahme des Pflegerisikos im Alter: Welche Rolle kommt der Familie und der sozialen Sicherheit zu, in: Internationale Revue für soziale Sicherheit, Vol. 50, No. 1, 25-45

Higgins, J. (1987): 'States of Welfare' – Comparative Analysis in Social Policy, Oxford: Oxford University Press

Himmelweit, S. (1995): The Discovery of "Unpaid Work": The Social Consequences of the Expansion of "Work", in: Feminist Economics, Vol. 1, No. 2, 1-19

Holzmann, A., Österle, A. (1996): Impact of Payments for Care on the Labour-Market Position of Informal Care-Givers, Paper presented at the 30th Annual SPA Conference, Sheffield

Hooyan, N.R. (1990): Women as Caregivers of the Elderly. Implications for Social Policy and Practice, in: Biegel, D.E., Blum, A. (Eds.): Aging and Caregiving. Theory, Research, and Policy, London: Sage

Hoskins, I. (1993): Combining Work and Care for the Elderly: An Overview of the Issues, in: International Labour Review, Vol. 132, No. 3, 347-369

Hugman, R. (1994): Ageing and the Care for Older People in Europe, London: Macmillan

Hutten, J.B.F. (1996a): Home Care in Italy, in: Hutten, Kerkstra (1996)

Hutten, J.B.F. (1996b): Home Care in the United Kingdom, in: Hutten, Kerkstra (1996)

Hutten, J.B.F., Kerkstra, A. (Eds.) (1996): Home Care in Europe. A Country-Specific Guide to its Organization and Financing, Aldershot: Arena

ISTAT (1997): Anziani in Italia, Bologna: Il Mulino

Jackson, W.A. (1998): The Political Economy of Population Ageing, Cheltenham: Edward Elgar

Jacobs, L.A. (1993): Realizing Equal Life Prospects: The Case for a Perfectionist Theory of Fair Shares, in: Drover, G., Kerans, P. (Eds.): New Approaches to Welfare Theory, Aldershot: Edward Elgar

Jacobzone, S. (1999): Ageing and Care for Frail Elderly Persons: An Overview of International Perspectives, OECD Labour Market and Social Policy Occasional Papers No. 38, Paris

Jacobzone, S., Cambois, E., Chaplain, E., Robine, J.-M. (1999): The Health of Older Persons in OECD Countries: Is it Improving Fast Enough to Compensate for Population Ageing?, OECD Labour Market and Social Policy Occasional Papers No. 37, Paris

Jamieson, A. (Ed.) (1991): Home Care for Older People in Europe. A Comparison of Policies and Practices, Oxford: Oxford University Press

Jamieson, A., Illsley, R. (Eds.) (1990): Contrasting European Policies for the Care of Older People, Aldershot: Avebury

Jani Le-Bris, H. (1993): Family Care of Older People in the European Community, Dublin: European Foundation for the Improvement of Living and Working Conditions

Janoski, T., Hicks, A.M. (Eds.) (1994a): The Comparative Political Economy of the Welfare State, Cambridge: Cambridge University Press

Janoski, T., Hicks, A.M. (1994b): Methodological Innovations in Comparative Political Economy. An Introduction, in: Janoski, Hicks (1994a)

Jones, C. (1985): Patterns of Social Policy. An Introduction to Comparative Analysis, London: Tavistock

Jordan, B. (1996): A Theory of Poverty and Social Exclusion, Cambridge: Polity Press

Joshi, H. (1995): The Labour Market and Unpaid Caring: Conflict and Compromise, in: Allen, Perkins (1995)

Kalisch, D.W., Aman, T., Buchele, L.A. (1998): Social and Health Policies in OECD Countries: A Survey of Current Programmes and Recent Developments. Labour Market and Social Policy Occasional Papers No. 33, Paris: OECD

Kane, R.A. (1995): Expanding the Home Care Concept. Blurring Distinctions among Home Care, Institutional Care, and Other Long-Term-Care Services, in: The Milbank Quarterly, Vol. 73, No. 2, 161-186

Kass, D. (1987): Economies of Scale and Scope in the Provision of Home Health Services, in: Journal of Health Economics, Vol. 6, 129-146

Keigher, S.M. (1997): Austria's New Attendance Allowance: A Consumer-Choice Model of Care for the Frail and Elderly, in: International Journal of Health Services, Vol. 27, No. 4, 753-765

Kemper, P. (1992): The Use of Formal and Informal Home Care by the Disabled Elderly, in: Health Services Research, Vol. 27, No. 4, 421-451

Kemper, P., Applebaum, R., Harrigan, M. (1987): Community Care Demonstrations: What Have We Learned?, in: Health Care Financing Review, Vol. 8, No. 4, 87-100

Kerkstra, A. (1996): Home Care in The Netherlands, in: Hutten, Kerkstra (1996)

Kerkstra, A., Hutten, J.B.F. (1996): A Cross-National Comparison of Home Care in Europe. Summary of the Findings, in: Hutten, Kerkstra (1996)

Klein, T. (1996): Determinants of Institutionalization in Old Age, in: Eisen, Sloan (1996)

Knapp, M. (1984): The Economics of Social Care, London: Macmillan

Knijn, T., Kremer, M. (1997): Gender and the Caring Dimension of Welfare States: Toward Inclusive Citizenship, in: Social Politics, Vol. 4, No. 3, 328-361

Kobayashi, R. (1997): Developing health and long-term care for a more aged society, in: OECD (1997)

Kohl, J. (1993): Der Wohlfahrtsstaat in vergleichender Perspektive. Anmerkungen zu Esping-Andersens 'The Three Worlds of Welfare Capitalism', in: Zeitschrift für Sozialreform, Vol. 39, No. 2, 67-82

Kohn, M.L. (1989): Introduction, in: Kohn, Melvin L. (Ed.): Cross-National Research in Sociology, Newbury Park: Sage

Kolm, S.-C. (1996): Modern Theories of Justice, Cambridge: The MIT Press

Kolm, S.-C. (1997): Justice and Equity, Cambridge: MIT Press (originally published 1971 in french)

Laing, W. (1993): Financing Long-Term Care. The Crucial Debate, London: ACE Books

Lambert, P.J. (1989): The Distribution and Redistribution of Income. A Mathematical Analysis, Oxford: Basil Blackwell

Lamura, G., Melchiorre, M.G., Tarabelli, D., Ciarrocchi, S., Quattrini, S., Mengani, M. (1999): Elderly in Italy: Policy Implications Coming from Current Socio-Demographic Trends and Recent Empirical Findings on Family Care-Giving, Paper presented at the International Seminar "The Consequences of Population Aging for Society", CEPS/INSTEAD, Differdange, July 16-23, 1999

Langan, M. (1998): The Contested Concept of Need, in: Langan, M. (Ed.): Welfare: Needs, Rights and Risks, London: Routledge

Langan, M., Ostner, I. (1991): Gender and Welfare. Towards a Comparative Framework, in: Room, G. (Ed.): Towards a European Welfare State, Bristol: SAUS

Le Grand, J. (1982): The Strategy of Equality. Redistribution and the Social Services, London: George Allen & Unwin

Le Grand, J. (1991): Equity and Choice. An Essay in Economics and Applied Philosophy, London: Harper Collins

Leat, D. (1990): For Love and Money. The Role of Payment in Encouraging the Provision of Care, London: Joseph Rowntree Foundation

Leat, D., Perkins, E. (1998): Juggling and Dealing: The Creative Work of Care Package Purchasing, in: Social Policy & Administration, Vol. 32, No. 2, 166-181

Leat, D., Ungerson, C. (1994): Payments for Care: The Case of Britain, in: Evers, Pijl, Ungerson (1994)

Lee, T. (1996): The Search for Equity. The Funding of Additional Educational Needs under LMS, Aldershot: Avebury

Leibfried, S. (1993): Towards a European Welfare State? On Integrating Poverty Regimes into the European Community, in: Jones, Catherine

(Ed.): New Perspectives on the Welfare State in Europe, London: Routledge

Leichsenring, K. (1999): Social Protection for Dependency in Old Age in Austria. National Report Series for the Social Protection for Dependency in Old Age in the 15 EU Member States and Norway Project, Leuven: HIVA

Lerner, M.J., Mikula, G. (Eds.) (1994): Entitlement and the Affectional Bond. Justice in Close Relationships, New York: Plenum

Lesemann, F., Martin, C. (Eds.) (1993): Home-Based Care, the Elderly, the Family, and the Welfare State: An International Comparison, Ottawa: University of Ottawa Press

Leutz, W. (1986): Long-Term Care for the Elderly: Public Dramas and Private Realities, in: Inquiry, Vol. 23, No. 2, 134-140

Levorato, A., Rozzini, R., Trabucchi, M. (1994): I costi della vecchiaia. L'assistenza sanitiaria agli anziani negli anni '90, Bologna: Il Mulino

Lewis, J. (1992): Gender and the Development of Welfare Regimes, in: Journal of European Social Policy, Vol. 2, No. 3, 159-173

Lewis, J. (1994): Choice, Needs and Enabling: The New Community Care, in: Oakley, A., Williams, A.S. (Eds.): The Politics of the Welfare State, London: UCL Press

Longo, F. (1997): I servizi per gli anziani in Italia: una rete di aziende in un gioco competitivo a somma negative. Ipotesi per un nuovo sistema di relazione, in: Mecosan, Vol. VI, No. 23, 51-65

Mannion, R., Smith, P. (1998): How Providers are Chosen in the Mixed Economy of Community Care, in: Bartlett, Will, Roberts, Jennifer A., Le Grand, Julian (Eds.): A Revolution in Social Policy. Quasi-Market Reforms in the 1990s, Bristol: Polity Press

Manton, K.G. (1982): Changing Concepts of Morbidity and Mortality in the Elderly Population, in: Milbank Memorial Foundation Quarterly / Health and Society, Vol. 60, 183-244

Manton, K.G., Corder, L.S. (1998): Forecasts of Future Disabled and Institutionalised US Populations 1995 to 2040, in: Marmor, T.R., De Jong, P.R. (Eds.): Ageing, Social Security and Affordability, Aldershot: Ashgate

Manton, K.G., Corder, L.S., Stallard, E. (1993): Estimates of Change in Chronic Disability and Institutional Incidence and Prevalence Rates in the U.S. Elderly Population from the 1982, 1984, and 1989 National Long-Term Care Survey, in: Journal of Gerontology, Vol. 48, No. 4, 153-166

Martin, C. (Ed.) (2001): Les personnes âgées dépendantes. Quelles politiques en Europe?, Rennes: Presses de l'Université de Rennes et Édition de l'Ecole Nationale de la Santé Publique

Martin, S., Smith, P.C. (1999): Rationing by Waiting Lists: An Empirical Investigation, in: Journal of Public Economics, Vol 71, 141-164

Mayhew, L. (2000) Health and Elderly Care. Expenditure in an Aging World. IIASA Research Report RR-00-21, Laxenburg: International Institute for Applied Social Sciences

McKay, N.L. (1988): An Econometric Analysis of Costs and Scale Economies in the Nursing Home Industry, in: The Journal of Human Resources, Vol. 23, No. 1, 57-75

Mengani, M., Lamura, G., Melchiorre, M.G. (Eds.) (1999): L'assistenza famigliare agli anziani. La situazione nel Commune di Senigallia, Ancona: il lavoro editoriale

Mikula, G. (1998): Division of Household Labor and Perceived Justice: A Growing Field of Research, in: Social Justice Research, Vol. 11, No. 3, 214-241

Millar, J., Warman, A. (1996): Defining Family Obligations in Europe, London: Family Policy Studies Centre

Miller, D. (1992): Distributive Justice: What the Poeple Think, in: Ethics, Vol. 102, No. 3, 555-593

Mishra, R. (1981): Society and Social Policy, Basingstoke: Macmillan

Montada, L., Lerner, M.J. (Eds.) (1996): Current Societal Concerns about Justice, New York: Plenum Press

Montanelli, R. (1998): L'assistenza agli anziani in ADI e in RSA: confronto tra politiche alternative e analisi dei costi, Mecosan, Vol VII, No. 28, 49-59

Moody, H.P. (Ed.) (1998): Aging. Concepts & Controversies. 2nd Edition, Thousand Oaks: Pine Forge Press

Mooney, G. (1992): Economics, Medicine and Health Care. 2nd Edition, New York: Harvester Wheatsheaf

Morelli, A. (1998): Poche regioni staccano l'assegno per le famiglie che assistono l'anziano, in: Agenzia Sanitaria Italiana, No. 18, 38-39

Morris, J. (1993): Independent Lives: Community Care and Disabled People, London: Macmillan

Mueller, D.C. (1989): Public Choice II, Cambridge: Cambridge University Press

Musgrave, R.A. (1959): The Theory of Public Finance, New York: McGraw Hill

Musgrave, R.A., Musgrave, P.B. (1989): Public Finance in Theory and Practice. 5th Edition, New York: McGraw Hill

Naegele, G., Reichert, M. (Eds.) (1998): Vereinbarkeit von Erwerbstätigkeit und Pflege. Nationale und internationale Perspektiven I, Hannover: Vincentz Verlag

Naegele, G., Reichert, M. (Eds.) (1999): Vereinbarkeit von Erwerbstätigkeit und Pflege. Nationale und internationale Perspektiven II, Hannover: Vincentz Verlag

Neal, M.B., Chapman, N.J., Ingersoll-Dayton, B., Emlen, A.C. (1993): Balancing Work and Caregiving for Children, Adults, and Elderly, Newbury Park: Sage

Netten, A., Davies, B. (1990): The Social Production of Welfare and Consumption of Social Services, in: Journal of Public Policies, Vol. 10, No. 3, 331-347

Nocera, S., Zweifel, P. (1996): Women's Role in the Provision of Long-Term Care, Financial Incentives, and the Future Financing of Long-Term Care, in: Eisen, Sloan (1996)

Nocon, A., Qureshi, H. (1996): Outcomes of Community Care for Users and Carers, Buckingham: Open University Press

O'Connor, J.S. (1993): Gender, Class and Citizenship in the Comparative Analysis of Welfare State Regimes: Theoretical and Methodological Issues, in: British Journal of Sociology, Vol. 44, No. 3, 501-518

O'Connor, J.S., Orloff, A.S., Shaver, S. (1999): States, Markets, Families. Gender, Liberalism and Social Policy in Australia, Canada, Great Britain and the United States, Cambridge: Cambridge University Press

O'Donnell, O., Propper, C., Upward, R. (1993): United Kingdom, in: Van Doorslaer, Wagstaff, Rutten (1993)

OECD (1988): Ageing Populations. The Social Policy Implications, Paris: OECD

OECD (1994): Caring for Frail Elderly People. New Directions in Care, Paris: OECD

OECD (1996): Ageing in OECD Countries. A Critical Policy Challenge, Paris: OECD

OECD (1997): Family, Market, and Community. Equity and Efficiency in Social Policy, Paris: OECD

OECD (1998): Maintaining Prosperity in an Ageing Society, Paris: OECD

OECD (1999): A Caring World. The New Social Policy Agenda, Paris: OECD

OECD (2000): OECD in Figures, Paris: OECD

Okma, K.G.H. (1998): Die Pflegeversicherung in den Niederlanden, in: Sieveking, K. (Ed.): Soziale Sicherung bei Pflegebedürftigkeit in der Europäischen Union, Baden-Baden: Nomos

Okun, A.M. (1975): Equality and Efficiency. The Big Tradeoff, Washington: The Brookings Institution

Olshansky, S.J., Rudberg, M.A., Carnes, B.A., Cassel, C.K., Brody, J.A. (1991): Trading Off Longer Life for Worsening Health: The Expansion of Morbidity Hypothesis, in: Journal of Aging and Health, Vol. 3, 194-216

Orloff, A.S. (1993): Gender and the social rights of citizenship. The comparative Analysis of Gender Relations and Welfare States, in: American Sociological Review, Vol. 58, No. 3, 303-328

ÖSTAT (Ed.) (1999): Statistisches Jahrbuch für die Republik Österreich 1999 – 2000, Wien: Österreichisches Statistisches Zentralamt

Øyen, E. (Ed.) (1990): Comparative Methodology. Theory and Practice in International Social Research, London: Sage

Paci, P., Wagstaff, A. (1993): Italy, in: Van Doorslaer, Wagstaff, Rutten (1993)

Pacolet, J., Bouten, R., Lanoye, H., Versieck, K. (1999a): Social Protection for Dependency in Old Age in the 15 EU Member States and Norway. Synthesis Report, Brussels: Commission of the European Communities

Pacolet, J., Bouten, R., Lanoye, H., Versieck, K. (1999b): Social Protection for Dependency in Old Age in the 15 EU Member States and Norway. Statistical and Institutional Annexes, Leuven: HIVA

Pacolet, J., Bouten, R., Lanoye, H., Versieck, K. (2000): Social Protection for Dependency in Old Age, Aldershot: Ashgate

Parker, G., Clarke, H. (1997): Will You Still Need Me, Will You Still Feed Me? – Paying for Care in Old Age, in: Social Policy & Administration, Vol. 31, No. 2, 119-135

Pauly, M.V. (1990): The Rational Nonpurchase of Long-Term Care Insurance, in: Journal of Political Economy, Vol. 98, No. 1, 153-168

Percy-Smith, J. (Ed.) (1996): Needs Assessments in Public Policy, Buckingham: Open University Press

Pereira, J. (1993): What does Equity in Health Mean?, in: Journal of Social Policy, Vol. 22, No. 1, 19-48

Pesaresi, F., Simoncelli, M. (1999): Le RSA nelle regioni italiane: Tipologia e dimensioni, in: ASI, Anno VI, No. 1-2, 14-36

Phillips, J. (1994): The Employment Consequences of Caring for Older People, in: Health and Social Care in the Community, Vol. 2, No. 3, 143-152

Phillips, J. (1995): Working Carers. International Perspectives on Working and Caring for Older People, Aldershot: Ashgate

Pierson, P. (1994): Dismantling the Welfare State? Reagan, Thatcher and the Politics of Retrenchment, Cambridge: Cambridge University Press

Pijl, M. (1993): Care for the Elderly in the Netherlands: New Policies and Practices, in: Lesemann, Martin (1993)

Pijl, M. (1994): When Private Care Goes Public. An Analysis of Concepts and Principles Concerning Payments of Care, in: Evers, Pijl, Ungerson (1994)

Plant, R. (1998): Citizenship, Rights, Welfare, in: Franklin, Jane (Ed.): Social Policy and Social Justice, Cambridge: Polity Press

Portrait, F., Lindeboom, M., Deeg, D. (2000): The Use of Long-Term Care Services by the Dutch Elderly, in: Health Economics, Vol. 9, No. 6, 513-531

Pratscher, K., Stolitzka, B. (1999): Sozialhilfe und sonstige Sozialleistungen der Bundesländer, in: Soziale Sicherheit, Vol. 54, No. 4, 264-270

Priestley, M. (1999): Disability Politics and Community Care, London: Jessica Kingsley

Prisching, M. (1996): Bilder des Wohlfahrtsstaates, Marburg: Metropolis Verlag

Putterman, L., Roemer, J.E., Silvestre, J. (1998): Does Egalitarianism have a Future?, in: Journal of Economic Literature, Vol. XXXVI, No. 2, 861-902

Quah, E. (1993): Economics and Home Production. Theory and Measurement, Aldershot: Avebury

Rae, D. (1981): Equalities, Cambridge: Harvard University Press

Ragin, C. (1987): The Comparative Method. Moving Beyond Qualitative and Quantitative Strategies, Berkeley: University of California Press

Rawls, J. (1971): A Theory of Justice, Cambridge: Harvard University Press

Reichle, B. (1996): From Is to Ought and the Kitchen Sink: On the Justice of Distributions in Close Relationships, in: Montada, Lerner (1996)

Rhoades, J.A. (1998): The Nursing Home Market. Supply and Demand for the Elderly, New York: Garland Publishing

Rhodes, M. (Ed.) (1997): Southern European Welfare States. Between Crisis and Reform, London: Cass

Richards, M. (1996): Community Care for Older People. Rights, Remedies and Finances, Bristol: Jordan

RIS MRC CFAS (1998): Mental and Physical Frailty in Older People: The Costs and Benefits of Informal Care, in: Ageing and Society, Vol. 18, No. 3, 317-354

Rodgers, G., Gore, C., Figueiredo, J.B. (Eds.) (1995): Social Exclusion. Rhetoric, Reality, Responses, Geneva: ILO Publications

Roemer, J.E. (1986): Equality of Resources Implies Equality of Welfare, in: The Quarterly Journal of Economics, Vol. 101, No. 4, 751-784

Roemer, J.E. (1996): Theories of Distributive Justice, Cambridge: Harvard University Press

Roemer, J.E. (1998): Equality of Opportunity, Cambridge: Harvard University Press

Room, G. (1993): Observatory on National Policies to Combat Social Exclusion. Second Annual Report, Brussels: Commission of the European Communities

Room, G. (Ed.) (1995): Beyond the Threshold. The Measurement and Analysis of Social Exclusion, Bristol: Polity Press

Rostgaard, T., Fridberg, T. (1998): Caring for Children and Older People – A Comparison of European Policies and Practices, Copenhagen: The Danish National Institute of Social Research

Rothstein, B. (1998): Just Institutions Matter. The Moral and Political Logic of the Universal Welfare State, Cambridge: Cambridge University Press

Rowlands, O. (1998): Informal Carers. An Independent Study Carried out by the Office for National Statistics, London: The Stationary Office

Rubisch, M. (1998): Die Umsetzung der Pflegevereinbarung zwischen Bund und Ländern, in: Soziale Sicherheit, No. 12, 941-945

Rudda, J. (1998): Die Novelle 1998 zum Bundespflegegeldgesetz, in: Soziale Sicherheit, No. 12, 918-925

Sainsbury, D. (1996): Gender, Equality and Welfare States, Cambridge: Cambridge University Press

Saltman, R.B., Figueras, J. (1997): European Health Care Reforms. Analysis of Current Strategies, Copenhagen: Word Health Organisation

Sanmann, H. (Ed.) (1973): Leitbilder und Zielsysteme der Sozialpolitik, Berlin: Duncker & Humblot

Saraceno, C. (1997): Family Change, Family Policies and the Restructuring of Welfare, in: OECD (1997)

Scanlon, W.J. (1992): Possible Reforms for Financing Long-Term Care, in: Journal of Economic Perspectives, Vol. 6, No. 3, 43-58

Scherer, K.R. (Ed.) (1992): Justice. Interdisciplinary Perspectives, Cambridge: Cambridge University Press

Schmähl, W. (1992): Zum Vergleich von Umlageverfahren und kapitalfundiertem Verfahren zur Finanzierung einer Pflegeversicherung in der Bundesrepublik Deutschland. Studie im Auftrag des Bundesministerium für Familie und Senioren, Stuttgart: Kohlhammer

Schmähl, W., Rothgang, H. (1996): The Long-Term Costs of Public Long-Term Care Insurance in Germany. Some Guesstimates, in: Eisen, Sloan (1996)

Schmidt, M.G. (1998): Sozialpolitik. Historische Entwicklung und internationaler Vergleich. 2nd Edition, Opladen: Leske+Budrich

Schmidt, V.H., Hartmann, B.K. (1997): Lokale Gerechtigkeit in Deutschland, Opladen: Westdeutscher Verlag

Schneekloth, U., Müller, U. (2000): Wirkungen der Pflegeversicherung, Baden-Baden: Nomos

Schokkaert, E. (1992): The Economics of Distributive Justice, Welfare and Freedom, in: Scherer (1992)

Schuijt-Lucassen, N., Knipscheer, C. (1999): Social Protection for Dependency in Old Age in the Netherlands. National Report Series for the Social Protection for Dependency in Old Age in the 15 EU Member States and Norway Project, Leuven: HIVA

Schulz, E., Leidl, R., König, H.-H. (2001): Auswirkungen der demographischen Entwicklung auf die Zahl der Pflegefälle bis 2020 mit Ausblick auf 2050. DIW Discussion paper No. 240, Berlin: Deutsches Institut für Wirtschaftsforschung

Schulz-Nieswandt, F. (1991): Über das Verhältnis von Wirtschaftspolitik und Sozialpolitik. Sozialpolitik im System der Sozialwissenschaft, in: Zeitschrift für Sozialreform, Vol. 37, No. 9, 531-548

Schulz-Nieswandt, F. (1994): 'Ambulant oder stationär?' Eine sozialökonomische Analyse der Determinanten der Inanspruchnahme stationärer Altenpflege, Regensburg: eurotrans-Verlag

Schulz-Nieswandt, F. (1999): Optimale Versorgungspfade? Akutmedizin, medizinische Rehabilitation und Altenpflege in einem fragmentarischen Gesundheitswesen, in: von Konradowitz, H.-J., Schmidt, R. (Eds.): Sozialgerontologische Beiträge zur Neuorganisation und zu Perspektiven der gesundheitlichen und pflegerischen Versorgung im Alter, Regensburg: Transfer Verlag

Sen, A. (1982): Choice, Welfare and Measurement, Cambridge: MIT Press

Sen, A. (1985): Commodities and Capabilities, Amsterdam: North Holland

Sen, A. (1992): Inequality Reexamined, Oxford: Clarendon Press

Sgritta, G.B. (1994): The Generational Division of Welfare: Equity and Conflict, in: Qvortrup, J., Bardy, M., Sgritta, G., Wintersberger, H. (Eds.): Childhood Matters. Social Theory, Practice and Politics, Aldershot: Avebury

Shapiro, E., Tate, R. (1988): Who is really at risk of institutionalization?, in: The Gerontologist, Vol. 28, 237-245

Sievering, O. (1996): Pflegeversicherung. Allokative, meritorische und distributive Aspekte staatlicher Eingriffsmöglichkeiten, Frankfurt: Peter Lang

Sipilä, J. (1997): Comparative Research on Social Care Service Systems: How to Proceed?, in: Kautto, M. (Ed.): European Social Services – Policies and Priorities to the Year 2000, Helsinki: Stakes

Smeeding, T.M. (Ed.) (1987): Should Medical Care be Rationed by Age?, Totowa: Rowman & Littlefield

Smeeding, T., O'Higgins, M., Rainwater, L. (Eds.) (1989): Poverty, Inequality and Income Distribution in Comparative Perspective, London: Harvester Wheatsheaf

Spicker, P. (1995): Social Policy. Themes and Approaches, London: Prentice Hall

Spicker, P. (1996): Normative Comparisons of Social Security Systems, in: Hantrais, Mangen (1996)

Stiglitz, J.E. (2000): Economics of the Public Sector. 3rd Edition, New York: Norten

Sundström, G. (1994): Care by Families: An Overview of Trends, in: OECD (1994)

Taccani, P. (1999): Curare oggi, curare domani. Il care degli anziani, in: Prospettive Sociali e Sanitarie, No. 3/1999, 1-5

Tester, S. (1996): Community Care for Older People. A Comparative Perspective, Basingstoke: Macmillan

Tester, S. (1999): Comparative Approaches to Long-Term Care for Adults, in: Clasen (1999)

The Royal Commission on Long Term Care (1999): With Respect to Old Age. Long Term Care – Rights and Responsibilities. Chairman: Sir Stewart Sutherland, London: Stationary Office

Tietzel, M. (Ed.) (1998): Ökonomische Theorie der Rationierung, München: Vahlen

Tietzel, M., Müller, C. (1998): Warteschlangen und Wartelisten, in: Tietzel (1998)

Tilly, J. (1999): Consumer-Directed Long-Term Care: Participants Experiences in Five Countries, PPI AARP Issue Brief No. 36, Washington: AARP

Titmuss, R. (1958): Essays on the Welfare State, London: Allen and Unwin

Törnblom, K. (1992): The social psychology of distributive justice, in: Scherer (1992)

Twigg, J. (1990): Carers of Elderly People: Models for Analysis, in: Jamieson, Illsley (1990)

Twigg, J., Atkin, K. (1995): Carers and Services: Factors Mediating Service Provision, in: Journal of Social Policy, Vol. 24, No. 1, 5-30

Twigg, J., Grand, A. (1998): Contrasting Legal Conceptions of Family Obligation and Financial Reciprocity in the Support of Older People: France and England, in: Ageing and Society, Vol. 18, No. 2, 131-146

Ungerson, C. (1990): The Language of Care: Crossing the Boundaries, in: Ungerson, Clare (Ed.): Gender and Caring: Work and Welfare in Britain and Scandinavia, Hemel Hempstead: Harvester Wheatsheaf

Ungerson, C. (1993): Payment for Caring - Mapping a Territory, in: Page, R., Deakin, N. (Eds.): The Costs of Welfare, Aldershot: Avebury

Ungerson, C. (1995): Gender, Cash and Informal Care: European Perspectives and Dilemmas, in: Journal of Social Policy, Vol. 24, No. 1, 31-52

Ungerson, C. (1997): Social Politics and the Commodification of Care, in: Social Politics, Vol. 4, No.3, 362-381

Ungerson, C. (2000): Thinking about the Production and Consumption of Long-Term Care in Britain: Does Gender Still Matter?, in: Journal of Social Policy, Vol. 29, No. 4, 623-643

van Doorslaer, E., Wagstaff, A. (1993): Equity in the Finance of Health Care: Methods and Findings, in: Van Doorslaer, Wagstaff, Rutten (1993)

van Doorslaer, E., Wagstaff, A., Bleichrodt, H., et al. (1997): Income-Related inequalities in Health: Some International Comparisons, in: Journal of Health Economics, Vol. 16, No. 1, 93-112

van Doorslaer, E., Wagstaff, A., Janssen, R. (1993): The Netherlands, in: Van Doorslaer, Wagstaff, Rutten (1993)

van Doorslaer, E., Wagstaff, A., Rutten, F. (Eds.) (1993): Equity in the Finance and Delivery of Health Care. An International Perspective, Oxford: Oxford University Press

van Doorslaer, E., Wagstaff, A., van der Burg, H. (1999): The Redistributive Effect of Health Care Finance in Twelve OECD Countries, in: Journal of Health Economics, Vol. 18, No. 3, 291-313

van Oorschot, W. (1991): Non-Take-Up of Social Security Benefits in Europe, in: Journal of European Social Policy, Vol. 1, No. 1, 15-30

Wagner, C. (1996): Home Care in Austria, in: Hutten, Kerkstra (1996)

Walker, A. (1995): Integrating the Family into a Mixed Economy of Care, in: Allen, Perkins (1995)

Walker, A., Guillemard, A.-M., Alber, J. (1993): Older People in Europe: Social and Economic Policies. The 1993 Report of the European Observatory, Luxembourg: Commission of the European Communities

Walker, A., Maltby, T. (1997): Ageing Europe, Buckingham: Open University Press

Walker, L.C., Bradley, E.H., Wetle, T. (Eds.) (1998): Public and Private Responsibilities in Long-Term Care. Finding the Balance, Baltimore: The Johns Hopkins University Press

Walker, L.C., Burwell, B. (1998): Access to Public Resources: Regulating Asset Transfers for Long-Term Care, in: Walker, Bradley, Wetle (1998)

Walzer, M. (1983): Spheres of Justice, New York: Basic Books

Watson, E.A., Mears, J. (1999): Women, Work and Care of the Elderly, Aldershot: Ashgate

Weekers, S., Pijl, M. (1998): Home Care and Care Allowances in the European Union, Utrecht: NIZW

White-Means, S.I. (1997): The Demands of Persons with Disabilities for Home Health Care and the Economic Consequences for Informal Caregivers, in: Social Science Quarterly, Vol. 78, No. 4, 955-972

WHO (Ed.) (1980): International Classification of Impairments, Disabilities, and Handicaps, Geneva: World Health Organization

Wiener, J.M. (1996): Long-Term Care Reform: An International Perspective, in: OECD (Ed.): Health Care Reform. The Will to Change, Paris: OECD

Wiener, J.M. (1998): Jump Starting the Market: Public Subsidies for Private Long-Term Care Insurance, in: Walker, Bradley, Wetle (1998)

Wiener, J.M., Illston, L.H., Hanley, R.J. (1994): Sharing the Burden: Strategies for Public and Private Long-Term Care Insurance, Washington: The Brookings Institution

WIFO (Österreichisches Institut für Wirtschaftsforschung) (Ed.) (1996): Umverteilung durch öffentliche Haushalte in Österreich. Studie im Auftrag des Bundesministeriums für Finanzen, Wien: Österreichisches Institut für Wirtschaftsforschung

Wilensky, H. (1975): The Welfare State and Equality, Berkeley: University of California Press

Wilensky, H., Lebeaux, C.N. (1958): Industrial Society and Social Welfare, New York: Russel Sage

Williams, A. (1997): Need as a Demand Concept (with special reference to health), in: Culyer, Anthony J., Maynard, Alan (Eds.): Being Reasonable about the Economics of Health. Selected Essays by Alan Williams, Cheltenham: Edward Elgar

Wilmot, S. (1997): The Ethics of Community Care, London: Cassell

Wilson, T., Wilson, D. (Eds.) (1991): The State and Social Welfare. The Objectives of Policy, London: Longman

Wistow, G., Knapp, M., Hardy, B., Allen, C. (1994): Social Care in a Mixed Economy, Buckingham: Open University Press

Wolf, D.A., Soldo, B.J. (1994): Married Women's Allocation of Time to Employment and Care of Elderly Parents, in: Journal of Human Resources, Vol. XXIX, No. 4, 1259-1276

Wolfe, B. (1986): Health Status and Medical Expenditure: Is There a Link?, in: Social Science and Medicine, Vol. 22, 993-999

Young, H.P. (1994): Equity. In Theory and Practice, Princeton: Princeton University Press

Zweifel, P., Breyer, F. (1997): Health Economics, New York: Oxford University Press

Index

Milton Keynes UK
Ingram Content Group UK Ltd.
UKHW040058071024
449327UK00019B/652